The Truth About Chronic Pain Treatments

THE TRUTH ABOUT CHRONIC PAIN TREATMENTS

ISBN Number: 978-0-9966862-04

Morning Light Books, LLC

Delmar, NY

To contact the author,

cindyperlin@gmail.com

The Truth About Chronic Pain Treatments:

The Best and Worst Strategies for Becoming Pain Free

Morning Light Books
Delmar, NY

Cindy Perlin, LCSW

This book is dedicated to those who suffer needlessly from chronic pain

Contents

Introduction 1

Chapter 1: How Do We Know What Works?...................7

Chapter 2: Pharmaceutical Treatments 17

Chapter 3: Injections...43

Chapter 4: Surgical Treatments 51

Chapter 5: Mind/Body Treatments..............................61

Chapter 6: Manipulative and Body-Based Practices 87

Chapter 7: Nutritional Interventions..........................111

Chapter 8: Herbal Treatments 149

Chapter 9: Exercise 161

Chapter 10: Homeopathy...171

Chapter 11: Acupuncture...181

Chapter 12: Energy Healing 187

Chapter 13: Marijuana 195

Chapter 14: Low-level Laser Therapy.........................209

Chapter 15: Multidisciplinary Programs 217

Chapter 16: The Pain Treatment Parity Act 221

Notes...227

Introduction

If you suffer from chronic pain, you are not alone. Chronic pain affects 116 million Americans—more than those affected by diabetes, heart disease, and cancer combined.[1] Worldwide, more than 1.5 billion people suffer from chronic pain.[2] Back pain is the leading cause of disability in Americans younger than 45.[3] Chronic pain is also the leading cause of disability worldwide.[4]

In 2011, the Institute of Medicine estimated that pain costs the United States between $560 and $635 billion a year, including pain-related health care costs between $261 billion and $300 billion, and $297 billion to $336 billion in lost productivity.[5] The suffering is intense. Suicide risk is at least doubled in chronic pain patients.[6] Individuals with chronic pain die significantly earlier, from all causes, than those without chronic pain.[7] According to a 2011 National Academy of Sciences report, "The magnitude of the pain suffered by individuals and the associated costs constitute a crisis for America, both human and economic."[8]

Chronic pain is defined by the International Association for the Study of Pain as "pain that persists beyond normal tissue healing time, which is assumed to be 3 months."[9] Acute pain is a normal sensation triggered in the nervous system to alert you to possible injury and the need to take action. When pain is chronic, the pain signals keep firing in the nervous system, long beyond normal healing time. Or there may be an ongoing cause of pain, such as arthritis. Some people suffer chronic pain in the absence of any obvious past injury or evidence of body damage. Common chronic pain conditions include headache; low-back and neck pain; and pain from cancer, arthritis, or nerve damage.[10]

The high prevalence of chronic pain is a strong indicator that the prevailing methods of pain treatment are ineffective. Conventional treatments for pain rely heavily on the use of pharmaceuticals, taken orally or injected, and surgery. These treatments have not curbed the epidemic of chronic pain. In fact, as I will describe in this book, all available evidence suggests that pharmaceuticals and surgery have increased the suffering, disability, and death rate of chronic pain patients.

There are many effective treatments for chronic pain, including mind/body methods of treatment, exercise, nutrition, herbs, acupuncture, and bodywork. Despite the magnitude of suffering by people in chronic pain, these treatments are largely ignored by physicians and, in many cases, are actively suppressed by the medical establishment: the Food and Drug Administration, the American Medical Association, health insurance companies, medical journals, and pharmaceutical companies. This suppression, which will be documented in this book, includes censorship of information, spreading of misinformation, refusal to fund research or treatment, failure to report positive research findings, and attempts to outlaw certain practices.

Pain is not caused by a pharmaceutical deficiency. Pain is rarely caused by a structural deficiency of the spine, even if one shows up on an MRI. Pain has many causes, including these common ones:

- Muscle weakness, stiffness, or spasm
- Inflammation
- Chronic tension caused by stress or unresolved emotional trauma
- Nutritional deficiencies
- Food sensitivities
- Toxins

Physicians Know Very Little About Pain Treatment

Your doctor is unlikely to be knowledgeable about pain treatment. According to a recent survey of the 104 US medical schools for which curriculum data were available, 20% of medical schools offered no pain education at all. Only four schools (3.8%) had a required course on pain. Information on the causes of pain and its treatment, if included at all, is usually covered in a more general required course that is not specifically focused on pain. Only 44 (42%) of the schools covered pharmacological pain management, and the average number of hours devoted to pharmacological pain management was 0.7. Only 37 (35%) of the schools addressed nonpharmacological pain management, including counseling/shared decision-making, conservative pain treatments, evidence-based complementary and alternative medicine, clinical psychology of pain, and rehabilitation of pain. The average number of hours devoted to nonpharmacological pain management was 1.1.[11]

The journals physicians rely on for ongoing medical education also fail to provide much information about pain treatment, especially about alternative treatments, as shown by the analysis of more than 10 years of articles[12] in some top medical journals, shown in Table 1.

■ TABLE 1. Prevalence of journal articles on pain and alternative medicine approaches to chronic pain, 2003 to mid-2014			
General medical journal	Number of articles	Number (%) of articles on pain	Number (%) of articles on alternative pain treatment
Journal of Pediatrics	7,787	31 (0.3%)	0 (0%)
Pediatrics	9,876	208 (2%)	5 (0.05%)
Journal of the American Medical Association	11,733	141 (1.2%)	6 (0.05%)
New England Journal of Medicine	16,528	90 (0.5%)	4 (0.02%)
Lancet	17,436	56 (0.3%)	19 (0.1%)
British Medical Journal	26,832	487 (1.8%)	40 (0.15%)

Even a pain specialist or a doctor who takes special interest in pain treatment and subscribes to medical journals focused on the subject will not learn much about nonpharmacological or nonsurgical treatments of pain. See Table 2 for an analysis of articles on alternative treatments for pain appearing in several top pain journals over a 10-year span.

TABLE 2. Prevalence of articles in pain journals that focus on alternative treatments 2003 to mid-2014		
Pain journal	Number of articles	Number (%) of articles on alternative pain treatment
European Journal of Pain	1,098	21 (1.9%)
Pain	300	18 (6%)
Journal of Pain	2,800	12 (0.4%)
Spine	7,381	87 (1.1%)

Physician conferences similarly offer few opportunities to learn about nonpharmacological and nonsurgical methods of treating pain.[13] An exception is seen in the conferences sponsored by the American Academy of Pain Management (AAPM) and its journal, *The Pain Practitioner*. The AAPM states that it is "the only professional pain management association that embraces an integrative model of care".[14] It's also probably the only professional organization where you will find MDs, chiropractors, psychologists, and naturopaths under one "roof."

Most physicians know they're not adequately prepared to treat chronic pain. Of 500 primary care physicians surveyed at 12 academic medical centers, only 34% reported that they felt comfortable treating chronic nonmalignant pain.[15] However, the competence of even these 34% is questionable. One study found no relationship between physicians' self-assessment of their knowledge and ability to treat pain and the quality of their treatment decisions.[16]

Physicians' knowledge gap regarding pain treatment can be easily exploited by pharmaceutical sales representatives. Often these salesmen and–women, trained and armed with marketing materials provided by their employers, are less than truthful about the benefits and risks of the drugs they promote.

This lack of physician preparedness is reflected in the experience of patients seeking treatment for chronic pain. In a study of their perception of their pain treatment, patients reported that primary care providers either did not appear to believe them or did not understand their suffering. Some providers were disrespectful. Many physicians spent very little time with patients and acted as though they were being kept from patients with "real" illnesses. Some patients reported that even when they asked about nonpharmacologic treatment, they were treated like addicts seeking drugs. These problems were reported by patients regardless of gender, ethnicity, age, language, socioeconomic status, and addiction history.[17]

For people in pain who want to get well, it's up to them to learn as much as they can about effective pain treatments and find ways to access those treatments most likely to benefit their individual situations. My goal in writing this book is to educate and guide chronic pain patients, their caregivers, and their health care providers in selecting the safest and most effective treatments.

Chapter 1

How Do We Know What Works?

In this book, I have presented the best information I could find on the promise and perils of available treatments for chronic pain. I have frequently cited research evidence, when available, about the treatments discussed. When it comes to research on the treatment of chronic pain, or any medical condition, there is considerable controversy, and many gaps. Health authorities often insist there is overwhelming proof for certain treatments while criticizing the lack of data for others. It is important for patients to understand the many factors that go into creating the body of medical evidence available, the degree of reliability of that information, and its applicability to their specific situation. I've included a brief discussion of research issues here to meet that need.

Evidence-Based Medicine

Since the early 1990s, there has been a push from many quarters for "evidence-based medicine" (EBM). According to the *British Medical Journal*, "The practice of evidence based medicine means integrating individual clinical expertise with the best available external clinical evidence from systematic research."[1]

According to EBM, all research is not created equal. The best evidence is considered to be meta-analyses of randomized clinical trials. A meta-analysis statistically pools results from many similar studies to draw conclusions about treatment effectiveness.

Second best, according to EBM, is evidence obtained from at least one randomized clinical trial. A randomized controlled trial is a study in which participants are assigned, by chance alone, to receive one of several interventions. One of these interventions is the comparison, or control. The control may be a standard treatment, a placebo (a sugar pill or fake treatment), or no intervention at all.

Double-blind randomized controlled studies are held in even higher regard. In a double-blind study, no one—patient, researcher, or any other results evaluator—knows which participants received which treatment. This ensures that no biases or expectations will influence results. Of course, double-blind studies are not possible when the treatment is anything more complicated than a pill, as practitioners administering the treatment must know what they're doing.

Nonrandomized prospective studies and observational studies are considered less conclusive. Expert opinion is considered the lowest level of evidence for making treatment decisions.[2]

In the EBM model, the evidence that comes from thousands of years of use and observation by indigenous healers across many cultures, such as in the use of acupuncture or herbs, is not considered valid, whereas results from a four- to eight-week study of a novel drug are given one of the highest rankings.

Flaws in the Research

EBM sounds good in theory, but its application to medical decision-making has left much to be desired. A 2014 article in the *Journal of Evaluation in Clinical Practice* reported that EBM has failed to achieve its main objectives: to improve health care outcomes and reduce health care costs.

Summarizing critics' concerns about EBM, authors Susanna Every-Palmer and Jeremy Howick wrote that one issue of major concern is that most studies available in medical literature are funded by parties that have a financial interest in the outcome, such as pharmaceutical companies. These entities manipulate the outcome of the research by their choice of issues studied and by manipulating the study design to favor their desired results. When the study still does not turn out as they had hoped, they fail to publish it and bury the results. Howick and Every-Palmer concluded that relying indiscriminately on industry-funded studies to make clinical decisions is like trusting politicians to count their own votes.[3]

Howick and Every-Palmer cited the evidence for selective serotonin re-uptake inhibitor (SSRI) antidepressants as an example. More than 1,000 randomized trials of SSRI antidepressants have been conducted, resulting in seemingly overwhelming evidence that they provide clinically significant benefits.[4] Doctors and patients were convinced that SSRI antidepressants (including Paxil and Prozac) worked. These blockbuster drugs posted global sales in 2011 of $11.9 billion.[5] SSRIs replaced older antidepressants and psychotherapy as the treatment of choice for depression. However, two independent analyses, published in 2008 and 2010, which included all published and unpublished studies on SSRI antidepressants, found that only favorable studies, and those that could be doctored to look favorable, were published. The pooled data from all studies showed that SSRIs are no more effective than placebo for the treatment of mild to moderate depression.[6,7]

A review of pharmaceutical company-funded studies that compared newer, atypical antipsychotics—touted as safer and more effective than the older generation—revealed that the drug produced by the company funding the study was found to be superior 90% of the time.[8] Studies were designed to make the study sponsor's drug appear superior by such means as setting the dose of the competing drug too low to be effective or so high that the side effects would be intolerable.[9]

Low-dose studies of natural treatments have also been funded by parties with an interest in discrediting competing treatments. This was the case with biofeedback, a treatment in which sensitive electronic instruments are used to measure the patient's physiology. That information is used to teach the patient to control her physiology and resolve her symptoms without medication. Biofeedback is used to treat chronic pain, headaches, high blood pressure, anxiety, insomnia, and many other conditions. The 1986 book *From the Ghost in the Box to Successful Biofeedback Training* documented key "errors" researchers made when conducting these studies.[10] One research methodology flaw involved an insufficient number of training sessions. Successful biofeedback treatment requires the mastery of complex skills, which is highly unlikely in the limited number of training sessions allowed by many studies.[11] Of 167 studies that took place before 1982 that used biofeedback to teach voluntary control of heart rate, 75% used only one to three sessions of biofeedback training.[12] Other research flaws included insufficient length of training sessions; lack of homework exercises (standard in most types of biofeedback treatment); failure to instruct subjects that the goal was to learn to control their responses; failure to provide adequate rationales, instructions, and coaching; use of a relaxation control group for comparison to biofeedback training (biofeedback is relaxation training); and failure to train to mastery.[13] While initially biofeedback generated a great deal of excitement, after these flawed studies were published, the interest substantially waned.

Failure to disclose the risks of pharmaceuticals is another issue with published research conducted by the drug's manufacturer. Pharmaceutical giants GlaxoSmithKline, Johnson & Johnson, Eli Lilly, and AstraZeneca have all been fined by the Food and Drug Administration (FDA) for hiding adverse effects of their products to make them more marketable.[14,15,16,17,18] More specific to pain research, Purdue Pharmaceuticals was charged by the federal government with a criminal count of misbranding the narcotic OxyContin (oxycodone), with intent to defraud, and falsely promoting it as nearly addiction-proof. I go into greater detail regarding the criminal proceedings and penalties faced by Purdue in the coming pages.[19]

In 2009, the world of pain medicine was rocked by the revelation that well-known anesthesiologist and researcher Scott Reuben had fabricated data in at least 21 published studies. Having received five research grants from Pfizer to study its drug Celebrex (celecoxib), Reuben went so far in some of the "studies" as to not bother enrolling patients and to make up all of the data, his findings naturally favoring Pfizer. These falsified findings influenced surgeons and the way they treated postoperative pain all over the world, affecting the care of millions of patients.[20] Reuben pled guilty to engaging in health care fraud. He was sentenced to six months in prison followed by three years of probation, a $5,000 fine, restitution of $361,932, and forfeiture of $50,000.[21] It's unclear how much harm was done to patients by Reuben's fabrications, but experts believe that implementation of his recommendations may have slowed surgical recovery.[22]

Another problem with the available body of evidence is that after research has been discredited, it is not retracted or labeled as fraudulent. The research studies remain available for the unwary to draw false conclusions regarding treatment safety and effectiveness.[23]

The prevailing research models are not appropriate for many alternative therapies, such as acupuncture or homeopathy, in part because treatments are not the same for every patient who presents for treatment of a specific condition. The choice of intervention is based on an assessment of the whole person, not just the presenting symptoms.[24] As a result, studies that give every patient with back pain, for instance, the same intervention are not valid measures of the effectiveness of these therapies.

Another related issue is the averaging of results in a study. What does or does not work for most people with a condition is not necessarily applicable to every individual in a study or in the overall population. Patients are individuals with different characteristics and combinations of symptoms, which might have different causes, who take different combinations of drugs. Treatment decisions that don't take individual differences into account are less likely to be effective and can cause harm.[25]

Bias in Funding

Another significant problem in evaluating evidence is that there is an uneven playing field when it comes to funding for research. Pharmaceutical companies, which can earn tens of billions of dollars in profit from patenting a single successful drug, can easily afford the hundreds of thousands of dollars it takes to conduct a drug study. Companies that sell foods, vitamins, or herbs that cannot be patented don't have that kind of money to invest in research that will benefit all companies selling a similar product. Health care providers who provide hands-on treatment—such as chiropractic, massage, or psychotherapy—are even more financially constrained, as they are limited to charging for their services by the hour. They cannot possibly generate enough extra income from their clinical work to fund a large research study.

Adding to the problem is the limited government funding available for medical research, and the fact that this funding rarely goes to those who challenge either the prevailing paradigm or those with power and influence.

The Case of Linus Pauling

Linus Pauling is considered by many to be one of the greatest scientists of the 20th century, one of the greatest chemists of all time, and the founding father of molecular biology. Pauling is the only person to have received two unshared Nobel Prizes. He won the Nobel Prize for Chemistry in 1954 and the Nobel Peace Prize in 1962. Among his many other prestigious awards is the National Medal of Science, presented to him by President Gerald Ford in 1975.

After Pauling obtained promising results in a small study he conducted of high-dose vitamin C for treating cancer, he applied five times for grants from the National Cancer Institute (NCI) to continue his work and was turned down every time.[26] Instead, the NCI funded a study of vitamin C in the treatment of cancer at the Mayo Clinic in 1979. Charles Moertel, an outspoken critic of Pauling, conducted a double-blind study intended to disprove Pauling's conclusions. Moertel's study deviated in important ways from Pauling's successful one, in part by failing to start patients off with 10 days of intravenous vitamin C and providing vitamin C for only two and a half months instead of continuing to administer it throughout the life of the patient. When Moertel's work failed to replicate Pauling's findings, Moertel was given widespread media coverage, and vitamin C therapy for cancer was pronounced a failure.[27]

The Case of Bessel van der Kolk

The same type of bias in funding still prevails. Bessel van der Kolk is an internationally renowned psychiatrist, trauma expert, and brain researcher. He is currently medical director of the Trauma Center affiliated with the Justice Resource Institute in Brookline, Massachusetts, and professor of psychiatry at Boston University Medical School. One of the first post-traumatic stress disorder (PTSD) researchers, van der Kolk conducted one of the first studies on Prozac (fluoxetine).

In recent years, he has come to recognize the limitations of pharmaceuticals in treating mental disorders and has remained open-minded about finding novel therapies to treat complex psychological trauma. Van der Kolk is very impressed by the results being obtained with neurofeedback (also known as brain wave biofeedback) in the treatment of PTSD. In particular, he is astounded by results with individuals who were repeatedly neglected and abused as children, a very difficult population to treat successfully. His repeated efforts to secure funding for a study of neurofeedback for traumatized children were unsuccessful. He is currently raising funds for his study through a crowdfunding website.[28]

Biases By and Against Journals

If a researcher of an alternative medical treatment is, despite all obstacles, successful at completing a research study that shows favorable results, he might have great difficulty getting a mainstream medical journal to publish the study. Medical journals rely heavily on pharmaceutical advertising to stay in business—and they don't want to upset their advertisers. The journal willing to print the results of the study might so offend the powers that be that the National Library of Medicine refuses to index it.

Andrew Saul, PhD, reported that the National Library of Medicine refuses to index the *Journal of Orthomolecular Medicine*, of which Saul is assistant editor, on MEDLINE, the number-one search tool for medical knowledge used by doctors and researchers. The National Library of Medicine, established by the US government in 1836, is the world's largest medical library. Its goal is to "collect, organize and make available biomedical literature to advance medical science and improve public health." One way the library does this is through its MEDLINE database, which it describes as "a huge database of over 17 million references to articles published in more than 5,200 current biomedical journals from the United States and over 80 foreign countries."

Saul further said:

> The *Journal of Orthomolecular Medicine* is peer reviewed and has been published for 41 years, so why isn't it indexed by MEDLINE? It has a review board of medical doctors and university and hospital-based researchers. Since 1967, it has published over 600 papers by renowned authors, including Nobel Prize winner Linus Pauling. According to MEDLINE, it is not included because it hasn't been scored high enough by their evaluation panel. I think that it is because they don't like what it said. In my opinion, they don't like the message. They do not want the public to have access to articles written by doctors for other doctors that are positive on megavitamin therapy because it is generally believed that drug medicine is the way that people should be cured. . . . [The decision on what journals to index is made by an unelected committee at the National Library of Medicine.] They decide what the taxpayer has access to. I don't think that a public library should censor, and the National Library of Medicine is a public library.[29]

Another important journal not indexed by MEDLINE is the *Journal of Neurotherapy,* which is published by the International Society for Neurofeedback and Research (ISNR). Neurofeedback, a therapy that teaches individuals to alter their brain activity to improve their health and functioning, has shown very positive results, both clinically and in research studies, regarding many treatment-resistant conditions, including chronic pain. The *Journal of Neurotherapy* is the only journal devoted exclusively to this field.

So what is a patient to do when faced with so much uncertainty? The most prudent path is to critically evaluate all the available evidence to the extent possible and start with the safest options first. I have written this book to help you with that.

Although researchers will argue it is not scientific, patients themselves provide another good source of information on real patient outcomes with pharmaceuticals. The websites www.askapatient.com and www.rxisk.com feature patients' posts on their positive and negative experiences with prescription drugs, searchable by drug name. . You can decide for yourself whether the possible benefits are worth the risks. Then you can consider other options, including those you will find in this book.

CHAPTER 2
Pharmaceutical Treatments

Pharmaceuticals are the most commonly used type of treatment in the United States for chronic pain. This includes both prescription and nonprescription drugs of various types, including nonsteroidal anti-inflammatory drugs (NSAIDs, such as aspirin, ibuprofen, naproxen, and Celebrex); steroids; opioids (also known as narcotics, opioids include morphine, methadone, fentanyl, oxycodone, and hydrocodone); anticonvulsants, such as Neurontin; and antidepressants (including the older tricyclics and the newer SSRIs). These pharmaceuticals tend to be limited in their effects on chronic pain and pose significant risks, as I will describe below.

Opioids

Americans are only 4.6% of the world's population but use 80% of the world's opioid supply. This is due, at least in part, to a recent concerted campaign in the United States to address the so-called undertreatment of pain.[1] The medical response to this "undertreatment" almost exclusively takes the form of treatment with narcotics. Between 1997 and 2006, the use of prescription narcotics skyrocketed. Hydrocodone use increased by 244%, the use of methadone increased 1177%, and the use of oxycodone increased 732%.[2]

Numerous literature reviews have concluded that there is weak, limited, or lacking evidence of effectiveness for the use of any opioid, including morphine, fentanyl, oxycodone, methadone, and hydrocodone, in the treatment of chronic pain.[3,4] Other studies have indicated that use of these drugs does not improve the quality of life in chronic pain patients.[5]

Opioid use has been associated with increased disability, medical costs, and subsequent surgery. One study found that prescription of opioids for low-back pain resulted in increased overall health care costs.[6] Other studies have shown increased duration of disability under workers' compensation for those who were prescribed opioids compared to those who were not,[7,8] and that the risk of surgery was three times greater for those who received early prescriptions for opioids than for those who did not.[9] A study in Denmark found that chronic pain patients who took opioids had worse pain, higher health care costs, and lower activity levels than similar patients not using opioids. The authors noted that opioid usage was significantly associated with reporting of moderate/severe or very severe pain, poor self-rated health, not being employed, higher use of health care services, and poorer quality of life. The researchers concluded that opioids failed to meet any of the goals of chronic pain management.[10]

A systematic review of opioids for the treatment of low-back pain by the Cochrane Database—a worldwide network of independent researchers, health care professionals, patients, and others—found that the few trials that compared opioids to NSAIDs or antidepressants showed no differences in outcomes for pain or function.[11]

Addiction and Abuse of Opioids

The disorder known as addiction results from continued use of a substance or engagement in an activity that may initially be rewarding but eventually becomes compulsive and interferes with work, relationships, or health. Opioids are highly addictive.

The problem of opioid addiction has received increasing attention in recent years, in the medical profession and in the media. Deaths from opioid overdose now exceed deaths from illegal street drugs. Prescription painkiller overdoses tripled in the United States between 1999 and 2008, killing nearly 15,000 people in 2008.[12] Nearly half a million emergency department visits in 2009 resulted from people misusing or abusing prescription painkillers.[13]

In 2010, enough prescription painkillers were prescribed to medicate every American adult around the clock for a month. Although most of these pills were prescribed for a medical purpose, many ended up in the hands of people who misused or abused them. Also in 2010, about 12 million Americans aged 12 or older reported they had used prescription painkillers for nonmedical purposes in the previous year.[14] Nonmedical use of prescription painkillers costs health insurers up to $72.5 billion annually in direct health care costs.[15]

It's not only nonmedical users of opioids who are getting addicted. Patients prescribed drugs for pain also become addicted. Chronic pain and addiction often overlap. One study found that 37% of patients in methadone maintenance and 24% of inpatients in drug treatment facilities reported severe chronic pain.[16] A study of unintentional overdose deaths during 2006 in West Virginia—which has the highest rate of overdose deaths of any state—found that about half of those who died had a medical history of pain treatment.[17] Estimates of the number of chronic pain patients addicted to painkillers vary widely, ranging from 2.8% to 50%.[18]

A report published in the *Washington Post* in 2012 concluded that drug companies falsified the study data they published to make it appear that the risk of addiction in pain patients was low. At the same time, drugmakers aggressively promoted their drugs to physicians as safe for chronic pain patients. As a result, physicians have liberally prescribed opioids to chronic pain patients, and almost 2 million Americans have become addicted.[19]

In the late '90s, Purdue Pharmaceuticals introduced what it touted as a nearly addiction-proof opioid: OxyContin. The company claimed that the drug's time-release formula would give patients steadier pain relief and allow them to avoid withdrawal. A promotional video from 1998 stated that the addiction rate for OxyContin users treated by doctors was less than 1%.[20] Its marketing was misleading enough that it led the federal government to charge Purdue with a criminal count of misbranding the drug "with intent to defraud and mislead the public." In its guilty plea, Purdue acknowledged that its promotional materials had contained misleading or inaccurate data and that its sales force had made claims unsupported by science that falsely downplayed the addiction risks.[21] While the company paid $635 million in penalties, it was a drop in the bucket; Purdue had revenue of $3.1 billion from OxyContin in 2010 alone.[22]

A survey of primary care providers conducted by Johns Hopkins Bloomberg School of Public Health and published in 2015 found that almost half incorrectly believed that pills with abuse-deterrent properties that prevented them from being crushed were less addictive than those without this abuse-deterrent technology. They are, in fact, equally addictive. One-third of doctors wrongly believed that most painkiller drug abuse occurs through snorting or injecting drugs, whereas, in fact, drugs of abuse are most commonly taken orally. According to study author Dr. G. Caleb Alexander, "Doctors continue to overestimate the effectiveness of prescription pain medications and underestimate their risks, and that's why we are facing such a public health crisis."[23]

Being rich and famous and having access to the "best" doctors doesn't prevent prescription painkiller addiction or death.

Michael Jackson

In June 2009, Michael Jackson, the "King of Pop," died from a drug overdose. Jackson's lifelong friend and biographer J. Randy Taarborrelli wrote after his death that Jackson was under medical supervision for severe chronic pain from back and knee problems, burns that he suffered while filming a commercial, complications from plastic surgery, and a host of other medical problems. He was addicted to painkillers, all prescribed by his physicians. Jackson believed he couldn't survive without the drugs that eventually killed him.[24] The precipitating cause of death was reported to be an injection of propofol, an anesthetic, by Dr. Conrad Murray. Jackson reportedly also regularly took two other painkillers, Dilaudid and Vicodin; the muscle relaxant Soma; the sedative Xanax; the antidepressant Zoloft; Paxil for anxiety; and the heartburn pill Prilosec. He was also reportedly being injected with the painkiller Demerol.[25] Jackson paid Murray $150,000 a month to travel with him and act as his personal physician. Murray had reportedly initially requested five million.[26] Murray was subsequently convicted of involuntary manslaughter.

Heath Ledger

Heath Ledger, the actor nominated for an Academy Award for his role in 2005's *Brokeback Mountain*, is another well-known figure who died from an accidental overdose of painkillers combined with other drugs. Ledger's death on January 22, 2008, stemmed from acute intoxication, according to the New York City medical examiner.

Heath Ledger (cont.)

Six drugs were found in Ledger's system: narcotic painkillers oxycodone and hydrocodone; antianxiety medications diazepam (the generic name for Valium); alprazolam (commonly known as Xanax); and temazepam, which is sold under the brand name Restoril and is often prescribed as a sleep medication; and doxylamine, an ingredient in some over-the-counter sleeping pills, also marketed in some nonprescription cold medicines that contain decongestants. The medical examiner reported that the combination of drugs, not any drug taken in excess, caused the death. Ledger's father reported that all of the prescription medications were "doctor prescribed."[27]

Philip Seymour Hoffman

Another celebrity who died of a narcotic-related overdose was well-regarded character actor Philip Seymour Hoffman, who, among many other accolades, won an Academy Award for his portrayal of the title figure in the movie *Capote*. Hoffman had reported that as a young man, he had been addicted to alcohol and drugs, including heroin, but had stopped using at the age of 22. One year before his death at the age of 46, Hoffman was admitted to a drug rehab program after his use of prescription painkillers led to a recurrence of heroin use. On February 2, 2014, he was found dead in his apartment from a heroin overdose.[28]

Patients with a history of abuse or physical or emotional trauma or who have PTSD are more vulnerable to becoming addicted to pain medication.[29] Current and past substance abuse also increases the risk for addiction to opioids used for pain management.[30] Use of opioids, despite the risk of addiction, is justified with the rationale that the stress produced by the "undertreatment" of chronic pain increases the likelihood of addiction.[31]

Many addiction specialists report that prescription painkillers now frequently act as gateway drugs to heroin use. Addiction specialist Jason Jerry estimates that about half of the heroin addicts seen by the Cleveland Clinic, where he works, first used prescription opiates. Jerry furthermore reports that the addiction often starts with a prescription for a legitimate medical condition. Once hooked on prescription painkillers, addicts find that heroin is cheaper and easier to obtain. Prescription painkillers also set off heroin cravings in recovering addicts.[32]

Dr. Andrew Kolodny, chief medical officer for the Phoenix House Foundation and president of Physicians for Responsible Opioid Prescribing, reported that areas with the highest rates of opioid or heroin addiction are often wealthier areas, where people have more access to medical care. In his experience, "almost all" the heroin users he has recently encountered started their opioid addiction with exposure to prescription painkillers.[33]

The Physiology of Addiction

People who become physically dependent on opioids (experiencing the need to keep taking the drug to avoid withdrawal syndrome) or addicted (experiencing intense craving for the drug or compulsive drug use) do so because of brain abnormalities created by chronic use of the drugs. When frequently exposed to increasing doses of opioids, the brain changes so that it functions normally when the drugs are present and abnormally when they are not. Over time, brain cells become less responsive to opioid stimulation, requiring larger doses to get the same effect (tolerance). The opioids initially suppress the brain's release of noradrenaline, which stimulates the body's alertness and ability to rise to demands. Gradually, the body adjusts by producing more noradrenaline, so that when the opioids are withdrawn, the body is overstimulated, producing jitters, anxiety, diarrhea, and muscle cramps. Chronic use of opioids also suppresses the brain's production of dopamine, a brain chemical linked to the ability to experience pleasure from normally enjoyable activities. As time passes, users begin turning to the drug not to achieve pleasure or pain relief but to avoid the extreme unpleasantness of withdrawal.[34]

Even More Opioids Enter the Market

Despite all the recent evidence linking prescription opioids to increasing rates of addiction and death, in October 2013, the FDA approved Zohydro ER, a new prescription opioid with five to ten times the potency of any other prescription opioid on the market. Unlike other prescription opioids, which combine the opiates with acetaminophen or aspirin, Zohydro is pure opioid. Zohydro also contains none of the abuse-prevention technology used in other prescription painkillers to prevent the drug from being crushed and snorted. Zohydro was approved by the FDA despite the recommendation of its own advisory committee, which voted 11 to 2 that the drug not be approved.[35] The drug hit the market in March 2014. Health care advocates and addiction specialists are petitioning the FDA to reverse their approval of the drug, and governors of at least two states, Vermont and Massachusetts, have moved to ban the use of Zohydro in their states.[36] Attorneys general from 28 US states have asked the FDA to withdraw its approval.[37] Regardless of the outcry, the FDA continues to defend its approval of Zohydro.

In May 2014, two California counties, hit hard by overdose deaths and the escalating health care costs related to prescription narcotics, filed a lawsuit against five narcotics manufacturers. The lawsuit alleges that the companies caused the counties' prescription drug epidemic with a deceptive campaign whose goal was to boost sales of potent painkillers such as OxyContin. The lawsuit accuses the drugmakers of violating California laws against false advertising, unfair business practices, and creating a public nuisance. Orange County District Attorney Tony Rackauckas reported that he decided to file the lawsuit to protect the public and "stop the lies."[38]

Despite the high level of protest against Zohydro, in July 2014, the FDA approved yet another high-dose extended-release opioid, Targiniq ER, which combines oxycodone with naloxone—an opioid agonist. The drug manufacturer claims that the addition of naloxone makes this drug abuse-resistant, failing to mention that this is true only if the drug is injected or snorted. Any benefit is lost, and the full dose of opioid released, if Targiniq is chewed. Meant to be taken once a day, Targiniq has twice the opioid dose of Zohydro. In violation of its own policy, the FDA avoided the embarrassment of ignoring the advice of a scientific advisory committee by neglecting to convene one to review approval of Targiniq.[39] The evidence for FDA approval of Targiniq was based on one 12-week clinical trial of patients who had moderate to severe low-back pain despite current use of less potent opioids.[40] Chewing Targiniq can result in overdose or death.[41]

Following the approval of Targiniq, and more generally in response to the FDA's continued irresponsibility in the face of an opioid epidemic, the Coalition to End the Opioid Epidemic petitioned the secretary of the US Department of Health and Human Services to "seek new leadership for FDA." A short time later, Rob Rappaport, director of the FDA's Division of Anesthesia, Analgesia, and Addiction Products, announced his "retirement."[42] For many a past FDA administrator, that phrase has signaled a shift to a lucrative career at one of the pharmaceutical companies whose bottom line the administrator helped increase.

This leadership change did not prevent the FDA, just a few months later, in November 2014, from approving yet another superstrength extended-release opioid, Hysingla ER. The FDA again did not convene an advisory panel before approving the drug. Manufactured by Purdue Pharma, Hysingla ER, is prescribed for once-a-day use, has 120 mg of hydrocodone, and claims to have abuse-deterrent features. Addiction experts, however, say that addicts know how to break down so-called abuse-deterrent products for oral use.[43] The FDA based its approval on one clinical trial of only 905 patients with chronic low-back pain.[44] The FDA-approved drug label includes a black box warning that states, "Instruct patients to swallow Hysingla ER tablets whole; crushing, chewing or dissolving Hysingla ER tablets can cause rapid release and absorption of a potentially fatal dose of hydrocodone."

Onus on the Physician

In the meantime, the medical community has turned its attention to promoting so-called "safe prescribing practices" for opioids. Prescribing physicians are told they are responsible for stemming the rising tide of addiction.

It can be extremely difficult for a physician to determine if a patient is an addict, whose drug-seeking behavior is an attempt to get high, or an individual truly in pain. This can be attributed at least in part to the fact that pain levels are subjective and often exist in the absence of obvious physical causes. Assessment of pain depends on the patient's report of its severity. On the other hand, addicts are well known for their manipulative skills and lies. When physicians, who are rarely trained in addiction, cannot distinguish between a patient who needs medication for pain relief and an addict trying to feed a habit, they are subject to loss of licensure and criminal prosecution.[45]

The Case of Dr. Frank Lizzi

Dr. Frank Lizzi was one such physician. Lizzi, board certified in hematology and internal medicine, practiced medicine for 32 years in Albany, New York, before surrendering his license in 2008, at the age of 69, rather than fight charges that he was overprescribing pain medication to his patients. Lizzi was a kind and compassionate physician, the old-fashioned kind who often spent more than an hour with a distressed patient and didn't charge those who couldn't pay. He was available to patients all hours of the day and night and even made house calls. When faced with charges of prescribing opioids to addicts, he could not afford to defend himself.

Lizzi reported that he had many patients who were in chronic pain, and many of them became addicted to opioids. These patients would tell him they were in terrible pain and needed more medication. Some, he referred to pain management specialists; and some came back to him saying they didn't want to be treated elsewhere. He referred other patients to drug detoxification units. Those patients didn't come back. Lizzi reported that it was hard for him to tell which patients were really in chronic pain, so for some, he would raise doses—a little. At one point, a patient told him that some of his other patients were selling their medication in the local park, but without identifying them by name. Another time the daughter of one of his patients told him he was overprescribing medication for her mother, and he cut back her dose. With the exception of making referrals for physical therapy, he was not prepared by his medical training to treat pain in any way other than with drugs. He ended his career teaching medical assistants.

Lizzi told me, "Maybe I should have been more mean" and refused pain medication to his patients. When the local newspaper reported Lizzi's troubles, his patients and some of his colleagues flooded the newspaper with calls and letters praising his caring and compassion and his willingness to go far beyond the call of duty. Lizzi died of cancer in April 2013, about five years after he lost his medical license. The stress of this experience no doubt contributed to his premature demise.

Lizzi and other physicians like him are often, like their patients, casualties of opioid treatment of chronic pain. Lizzi, in fact, got off easy. Doctors have become scapegoats in the war on drugs. Some doctors have been tried as drug kingpins and dealers and prosecuted for manslaughter when their patients misused the drugs they were prescribed and died of an overdose. These physicians, when convicted, are subject to the same draconian mandatory drug sentencing laws as violent individuals dealing illegal drugs. Under the Comprehensive Crime Control Act of 1984, the assets of suspected drug dealers, including MDs who treat pain with opioids, can be seized without hearings or trial; consequently, they are stripped of the assets they require to defend themselves.[46]

The Case of Dr. James Graves

In his 2008 book, *The Criminalization of Medicine: America's War on Doctors*, Ronald Libby recounts the stories of several physicians prosecuted for overprescribing, including Dr. James Graves, a family doctor in Pace, Florida, who specialized in pain management.

Graves was tried and convicted in 2002 for racketeering, drug trafficking, and manslaughter and received a sentence of 62 years in prison. Graves was the first doctor to be convicted of manslaughter as a result of prescribing painkillers to patients who died of an overdose. His case became a precedent for prosecutors to use against pain doctors across the country.

During his career, Graves worked on numerous occasions as a medical missionary in Ghana, Haiti, and India. He also served 17 years as a navy flight surgeon before being honorably discharged in 1994. After his discharge, Graves worked a series of temporary jobs before opening his own private practice in 1998. Graves was reported to the authorities for allegedly dealing drugs by a former employer, a chiropractor, who believed that Graves was violating a noncompete clause in his employment contract. As a result of this complaint, the government arrested Graves and closed down his practice in 2000. He had no income or savings and was forced to cash in a life insurance policy to post collateral for his bail bond. The court declared him indigent, and he was represented by public defenders. Prosecutors persuaded drug addicts facing extended jail time to entrap Graves and testify against him in exchange for more lenient sentences. Two doctors testifying for the defense stated that Graves's treatment of the patients who died was within the standard of care of medical practice in the United States and was for a legitimate medical purpose. None of the prosecution witnesses stated that Graves's treatment of the patients was wanton, reckless, grossly incompetent, or purposely homicidal. The prosecution failed to prove that he was medically negligent toward these patients, or even that he was the cause of his patients' deaths. Some of the deceased patients named in the trial were not even his patients or had died long after he stopped treating them. It was never proven that he accepted any money in return for drugs. Despite all of this, Graves was still convicted and sentenced to what amounts to life in prison.[47]

Cases such as Graves's allow the government to assert that it is doing something to address the problem of prescription drug addiction while allowing these highly addictive, very dangerous—but very profitable—drugs to stay on the market.

The risk of license revocation and prosecution coupled with the medical community's heavy reliance on narcotics to treat pain deters many physicians from specializing in pain medicine. This leaves many pain patients without viable treatment options.

Other Dangerous Side Effects

Prescription opioids pose many serious risks in addition to addiction, including negative effects on the immune system. Morphine and other narcotic drugs suppress antibody production along with the activity of three different types of white blood cells: T lymphocytes, B lymphocytes, and natural killer cells, which protect against cancer and bacterial and viral infections.[48, 49] The body's own natural painkillers, endorphins, have the opposite effect, enhancing immune response.[50]

Long-term use of opioids appears to decrease the body's production of its own natural painkillers.[51] This may be why, in the cruelest twist of all, some patients experience opioid-induced hyperalgesia (OIH), a condition in which patients taking opioids to control their pain become more sensitive to pain because of the opioid therapy.[52] This is different from tolerance, a well-known effect of opioids, which is the need to increase the dose over time to maintain pain relief. In OIH, increasing the dosage results in increased pain.[53] Consequently, long-term, or even short-term, use of opioids can actually increase rather than relieve chronic pain.[54]

Pharmacist Rob Gussenhoven noted that preoccupation with the problems of abuse, addiction, and overdose-deaths associated with opioids has diverted attention from the fact that once a chronic pain patient has been put on long-term opioids, he rarely recovers and his functioning deteriorates.[55]

Opioid users put others at risk as well. Opioids act on systems in the brain that affect alertness and driving ability, thus contributing to many motor vehicle accidents.[56]

Health care provider guidelines for prescribing responsibly include prescribing narcotic painkillers only when other treatments have not been effective for pain, according to the Centers for Disease Control.[57] Yet physicians rarely direct patients to nonpharmaceutical treatments for pain, instead going directly to their prescription pads. And although opioids entail more risks than other types of analgesics, physicians increasingly prescribe opioids before trying other drugs. In fact, one study found that prescriptions for opioids increased from 19.3% of back- and neck-pain patients in 1999 to 29.1% in 2010.[58] The opioid hydrocodone is now the most commonly prescribed drug in the United States.[59]

The casualness with which opioids are being prescribed is illustrated by my own experience with a dentist. After undergoing a tooth extraction as part of a dental implant procedure, I was handed a prescription—20 tablets, three refills—for Vicodin, a combination of hydrocodone and acetaminophen. The dentist did not ask me about my addiction history. He did not tell me the medication was a narcotic or that it could cause addiction. Because I knew about the drug, I decided not to take it and instead effectively managed pain from the procedure by taking three doses of ibuprofen over the next two days.

The American Academy of Pain Medicine (AAPM) is a society representing physicians who specialize in pain medicine. Their guidelines on the use of opioids for the management of chronic pain state:

> Pain should be diagnosed and treated in a comprehensive, systematic, collaborative, patient-centered fashion. Many strategies and options exist to treat and to manage chronic pain. Since chronic pain may have myriad causes and perpetuating factors, treatment strategies and options include interventional techniques, cognitive and behavioral methods, rehabilitation approaches, and the use of medications, including, where medically indicated, opioids.

Chronic opioid therapy (COT) should be reserved for those who have intractable chronic pain that is not adequately managed with more conservative or interventional methods. AAPM does not advocate opioids as a first-line therapy, but we believe that these medications may be useful if prescribed in a judicious manner as part of a logical progression of treatment.[60]

The group Physicians for Responsible Opioid Prescribing reports that there is little evidence that opioids are effective for chronic pain. The following is taken from its "Do's and Don'ts list":

DON'T initiate chronic opioid therapy (COT) before considering safer alternatives such as primary disease management, cognitive behavioral therapy (CBT), participating in pleasant and rewarding life activities, physical therapy, non-opioid analgesics and exercise.

DO screen patients for depression and other psychiatric disorders before initiating COT. Patients with depression and other mental health problems often present with pain problems. They may not know that mental health problems can contribute to chronic pain. These patients are at higher risk of opioid addiction. They may be better served by mental health treatment.[61]

In practice, few physicians, whether pain specialists or primary care doctors, adhere to these guidelines.

Nonnarcotic Pain Relievers: NSAIDs and Steroids

NSAIDs

A class of drugs called nonsteroidal anti-inflammatory drugs (NSAIDs) is used to treat mild to moderate pain, fever, and inflammation. NSAIDs work by reducing the levels of prostaglandins, chemicals produced by the human body that are responsible for pain and the fever and tenderness that accompany inflammation. NSAIDs block an enzyme, cyclooxygenase, which makes prostaglandins. This results in lower concentrations of prostaglandins, which causes a reduction in inflammation, pain, and fever.

The first NSAID in widespread use was aspirin. Aspirin's precursors, willow bark and other plant-derived resources, have been used to relieve pain and to reduce fever and inflammation for thousands of years. The current synthesized form of aspirin has been in use since the late 1800s. Aspirin use declined after the development of acetaminophen in 1956 and ibuprofen in 1962.[62] Acetaminophen (sold under the brand name Tylenol) became popular because it didn't cause gastric irritation, a side effect of aspirin.[63]

The FDA-required drug label lists the following serious adverse reactions to aspirin.

- Dysrhythmias
- Hypotension
- Tachycardia
- Cerebral Edema
- Coma
- Confusion
- Subdural or intracranial hemorrhage
- Seizures
- GI bleeding, ulceration, and perforation
- Hepatitis
- Reyes syndrome
- Pancreatitis
- Prolongation of prothrombin time
- Thrombocytopenia
- Acute Anaphylaxis
- Hypoglycemia
- Hyperglycemia
- Prolonged pregnancy and labor
- Stillbirths
- Lower birth weights
- Pulmonary edema
- Hearing loss
- Kidney insufficiency
- Kidney failure.[64]

The most frequent serious side effect of the NSAIDs aspirin and ibuprofen is gastrointestinal complication. Annually, 1% to 2% of people who regularly take NSAIDs, or 103,000 people, experience gastrointestinal complications serious enough to require hospitalization, at a cost of more than $2 billion, according to a study published in 2000. The same study estimated that 16,500 NSAID-related deaths occur each year in the United States among patients with rheumatoid arthritis and osteoarthritis.[65]

Paul

Paul Tick, a social worker in upstate New York, has suffered serious gastrointestinal consequences of NSAID use. When Paul was 21, he suffered a groin-muscle injury while lifting a garage door. The intense shooting pains in his groin lasted a year and then diminished to occasional pain. When Paul was in his 40s, the pain got worse, and he consulted many conventional and unconventional medical practitioners. After resisting medication use for many years, Paul started taking prescription ibuprofen at 800 mg on the advice of a physician. A few weeks later, Paul woke up feeling like he had the flu. He ended up in the emergency room with a diagnosis of ulcers in his esophaegus and stomach, a condition known as diffuse erosive gastritis. He was told there was an association between ibuprofen and this condition, but he wasn't told to stop taking the ibuprofen.

No one, Paul said, had ever warned him of any risks from taking ibuprofen. He was sent home with a prescription for Nexium, which he took for a day or two. Then he read the warning labels.

"It didn't seem right," Paul said. "The side effects of Nexium were the same as the symptoms I was having."

Paul (cont.)

He stopped taking all medication, but by this point his GI system was in terrible shape and he could not eat. Paul contacted a chiropractor who had treated him in the past, Dr. Joseph Olejak, who advised him to cook brown rice with extra water and drink the water; take herbs to prevent infections and heal his gut; and juice beets and cabbage.

Paul also consulted two holistic physicians, Dr. Ann Tobin and Dr. Sybil Stock, who advised him to juice additional fruits and vegetables to heal his gut. After a few days, Paul was feeling much better. After six weeks of juicing, he felt good. He kept up the juicing for about six months with gradually decreasing frequency.

Though Paul still has abdominal pain, he says he knows better than to treat it with drugs. He relies on deep tissue massage, chiropractic, and manual physical therapy to manage his pain.

More recently, cardiovascular risks of NSAIDs have become known. In July 2015, the FDA issued an advisory warning that nonaspirin NSAIDs—including ibuprofen, naproxen, and Celebrex (celecoxib)—increased the risk of heart attacks, heart failure, and strokes. The advisory stated that the risk increased with even small amounts of the drugs and that these drugs should be used sparingly for only short periods.[66] Years before the FDA warning, the National Library of Medicine and NIH warned:

> People who take nonsteroidal anti-inflammatory drugs (NSAIDs) (other than aspirin) such as ibuprofen may have a higher risk of having a heart attack or a stroke than people who do not take these medications. These events may happen without warning and may cause death.[67]

Acetaminophen, brand name Tylenol, is another potentially dangerous NSAID available over the counter and frequently used to treat pain. The most serious side effect of acetaminophen is liver toxicity, which can lead to liver failure and death. Acetaminophen hepatotoxicity, or liver toxicity, is now the most frequent cause of acute liver failure in many Western countries.[68] Data on the prevalence of this complication are very limited, with a conservative estimate by the drug's manufacturer of 213 deaths from liver failure because of acetaminophen overdose per year.[69] After several days or weeks of acetaminophen use at even the recommended doses, of up to 4 g daily, severe hepatotoxicity has been known to occur in individuals with chronic alcohol exposure.[70] Patients who are malnourished or have recently been fasting can experience liver failure at mild overdose levels of 10 g per day.[71] Although these risks have been known since the 1990s, few patients are aware of them.

Another thing few patients are aware of: the other drugs they are taking, either over the counter or prescription, may also contain Tylenol. It took until January 2014 for the FDA to issue an advisory to physicians that combination prescription painkillers containing more than 325 mg of acetaminophen per dose should no longer be prescribed because of the liver damage risk. Patients who have taken an overdose of acetaminophen will usually not manifest any symptoms until 24 to 48 hours after ingestion.

Several recent studies have suggested an association between the use of acetaminophen by women during pregnancy and the development of autism early in the life of their offspring.[72] Researchers believe the use of acetaminophen during early development may alter the immune system and increase the risk of autism in susceptible individuals.[73] Rates of autism began to escalate after parents were advised, in the early 1980s, to replace aspirin with acetaminophen to treat pain and fever in children.[74] There is also a strong association between the use of acetaminophen to treat pain and fever after a childhood vaccination and behavioral regression into autism shortly afterward. [75]

Based on concerns about gastrointestinal and other side effects from over-the-counter NSAIDs, a new class of prescription NSAIDs was developed in the 1990s, known as Cox 2 inhibitors. It was discovered that prostaglandins, which NSAIDs reduce to achieve their effect, come in two forms. Prostaglandins in which synthesis involves the cyclooxygenase-I enzyme, or COX-1, are responsible for maintenance and protection of the gastrointestinal tract. Prostaglandins in which synthesis involves the cyclooxygenase-II enzyme, or COX-2, are responsible for inflammation and pain. Aspirin and ibuprofen inhibit both types of prostaglandins, which leads to the GI side effects, while the Cox-2 inhibitors primarily affect the prostaglandins that cause inflammation and pain.

Cox-2 inhibitors Vioxx (rofecoxib) and Celebrex (celecoxib) were approved by the FDA in 1999 as supposedly safer NSAIDs. By 2004, Vioxx had been removed from the market after being linked to deadly side effects such as heart attack, stroke, kidney damage, and arrhythmia. Officially, up to 55,000 deaths have been attributed to the use of Vioxx,[76] and about 160,000 patients have been injured.[77] A federal lawsuit filed against Merck, the drug's manufacturer, included 50,000 claimants. Internal documents released during the lawsuit revealed that Merck knew of the cardiac dangers before its approval but did not provide this information to the FDA. Merck eventually settled these claims for $4.85 billion, also agreeing to pay $950 million in criminal fines and civil claims to the states and federal government for illegal marketing practices.[78]

The estimated 55,000 deaths attributed to Vioxx use might be a gross underestimate according to one investigator, Ron Unz, publisher of *The American Conservative.* Unz noticed that the year after Vioxx was removed from the market, the

United States saw the largest drop in its annual death rate in more than 60 years, despite the growth in the size and age of the US population. Upon further investigation, Unz found that the largest rise in the US mortality rates occurred in 1999, the year that Vioxx entered the market. Unz concluded it was possible that 500,000 Americans died from Vioxx in the five years it was on the market.[79]

The FDA was slow to remove Vioxx from the market, even after evidence of its risks became clear. The FDA requested that a similar drug, Bextra (valdecoxib), manufactured by Pfizer, be voluntarily removed from the market.

Another Cox-2 inhibitor, Celebrex (celecoxib), also manufactured by Pfizer, remains available. Studies have shown that it is no more effective at reducing pain than ibuprofen or other over-the-counter pain relievers.[80] And while Celebrex is also no better than other NSAIDs at protecting the stomach, Pfizer initially falsified data from its studies to make it seem safer.[81] A meta-analysis published in 2006 of Celebrex clinical trials lasting more than six weeks found that Celebrex more than doubled the risk of heart attacks compared to treatment with a placebo.[82] Long-term data on the cardiac safety of Celebrex are still not available. Pfizer announced a study of heart attack risks in 2005 that was not scheduled to be completed until 2014, when the patent for Celebrex was scheduled to expire.[83]

Despite its safety risks and lack of superior effectiveness to over-the-counter NSAIDs, almost 3 million prescriptions were written for Celebrex in 2013 in the United States, generating more than $2 billion in sales. Overseas sales generated another $1 billion.[84]

Steroids

Steroids, given orally or by injection, can reduce inflammation and pain and can slow joint damage in arthritis. Long-term use (months or years) is not recommended, as steroids can lead to the following:

- Osteoporosis
- Cataracts
- Weight gain
- Diabetes
- Muscle weakness
- Increased susceptibility to infection
- Hypertension
- Easy bruising
- Fragile skin

Steroids include Cortan, Deltasone, Meticorten (prednisone), and Medrol (methylprednisolone).[85] Even short-term use of steroids can cause a persistent elevated risk of bone death, also known as osteonecrosis, according to a 2011 study. In 92% of the cases, bone death was in the hip, but osteonecrosis of the knee and jaw were also reported. Use of steroids for as little as 30 days posed 3.8 times the risk of osteonecrosis. Use of steroids for one year led to 165 times the risk.[86]

Neurontin

Neurontin (gabapentin) was approved in 1993 solely for use with other drugs to control seizures in people with epilepsy. In 2004, Neurontin's manufacturer, Warner-Lambert, pled guilty to illegal and fraudulent promotion of unapproved uses for the drug, agreeing to pay more than $430 million in fines.

Neurontin was aggressively promoted for many conditions for which its effectiveness was not proven, including nerve pain, fibromyalgia, and migraine headaches.[87] This fine, a small fraction of Warner-Lambert's profits from the drug, did little to deter the company from continuing similar activities with Neurontin and other drugs. Warner-Lambert had been acquired in 2000 by Pfizer, a company that was fined $2.3 billion for illegal off-label promotion of their products in 2009.[88]

A 2014 Cochrane Collaboration review of the current evidence of Neurontin's effectiveness for chronic pain found 37 studies that had tested Neurontin against a placebo for four weeks or longer. There were adequate data to determine effectiveness for only two pain conditions: postherpetic neuralgia (chronic pain from shingles) and diabetic neuropathy. Neurontin helped 3 or 4 people out of 10 reduce their pain by at least 50%, compared to 2 out of 10 people on placebo. Sixty percent of Neurontin users had adverse effects.

The following side effects have been reported for Neurontin[89,90] :

- Dizziness
- Sleepiness
- Pain or swelling in the arms and legs
- Gait disturbance
- Increased risk of suicidal behavior and ideation
- Increased incidence of viral infections and fever
- Hypertension
- Migraines
- Anxiety
- Joint pain
- Abnormal vision
- In children: behavioral problems, hostility and aggressive behaviors, concentration problems, restlessness, and hyperactivity

Evidence of fraud, lack of evidence of effectiveness, and a high side-effect profile have done little to deter physicians from prescribing Neurontin, which posted sales of $2.3 billion in the United States in 2013.[91]

Antibiotic Treatment of Back Pain

In a study published in 2013 in the *European Spine Journal*, researchers at the University of Southern Denmark demonstrated how bacteria invade the sites of slipped discs, causing inflammation and harm to the surrounding vertebrae—a startling development. They found that almost half the patients in the study with slipped discs tested positive for infection, mostly by *Propionibacterium acnes,* the acne-causing bacteria. Another study by the same researchers tested an antibiotic combination treatment on 162 patients with slipped discs and signs of bone swelling. They found that treating the infection with antibiotics put an end to the back pain in 80% of the patients.[92]

Chapter 3
Injections for Pain

When oral medications fail and pain is localized, injections are often used to treat pain. A 2001 review reported "a lack of methodologically sound studies of surgery and injection therapies" and only limited (Level 3) evidence of effectiveness for any type of injections for pain relief.[1] Level 3 evidence generally means there are no controlled scientific studies supporting the treatment. A 2009 review of 15 randomized controlled trials of trigger point injections (TPI) to treat chronic musculoskeletal pain found that "the efficacy of TPI is no more certain than it was a decade ago as, overall, there is no clear evidence of either benefit or ineffectiveness."[2]

In 2013 an analysis was published of the use of epidural steroid injections in patients with lumbar spinal stenosis. Spinal stenosis is a narrowing of the spinal canal that results in neurological problems, including pain, numbness, tingling, tickling, or burning sensations, along with loss of motor control. The researchers found that patients who received the steroid injections showed significantly less improvement after four years than those who did not. Of the patients who subsequently underwent surgery, those who received the injections experienced a longer duration of surgery and a longer hospital stay.[3]

Patients with spinal stenosis who had epidural glucocorticoid (a type of steroid) injections with lidocaine (a local anesthetic) were compared with patients who had injections with lidocaine alone in a 2014 double-blind study.

Six weeks after injection, no significant difference in pain between the two groups was seen.[4]

Of patients experiencing spinal pain, those injected with saline solution did as well as those injected with steroids, and with fewer risks, according to a 2013 meta-analysis comparing epidural (spinal) steroid injections with injections of saline solution. Though the reason for this was unclear, the study authors speculated that it was either because of a placebo effect or because the injection of any fluids either has a detoxifying effect or stimulates the body's healing mechanisms.[5]

Risks of injections include superficial and deep infections. Other rare but serious complications include paralysis of the lower extremities, paraspinal abscesses, and meningitis.[6] On April 23, 2014, after decades of widespread use of steroid injections for pain, the FDA issued the following warning:

> Injections of corticosteroids into the epidural space of the spine may result in rare but serious adverse events, including loss of vision, stroke, paralysis, and death. . . . The effectiveness and safety of the drugs for this use have not been established, and the FDA has not approved corticosteroids for such use.[7]

An alternative type of injection, which uses plasma from the patient's own blood, appears to work better than steroid injections for long-term pain relief.[8]

A Safer Alternative

Another alternative type of injection, which seems safer and more effective, has been developed by Dr. Norman Marcus, a NYC physician who has devoted his professional life to the alleviation of chronic pain. Initially trained in psychiatry, Marcus subsequently trained in neurology, anesthesiology, and psychosomatic medicine. For the last 18 years, he has been on the faculty of the NYU Medical College in the departments of anesthesiology and psychiatry. He has authored two books and numerous journal articles on the treatment of chronic pain.

Marcus started several interdisciplinary pain clinics in New York City and one in England. When the New York interdisciplinary clinics met their demise—because of lack of insurance coverage (see a discussion of this issue in chapter 15)—Marcus opened his own clinic, the Norman Marcus Pain Institute (NMPI). The treatment program he personally developed focuses on muscles as generators of chronic pain. He invented an electrical device, the muscle pain detection device, that stimulates muscle tissue to help isolate those muscles with trigger points that are generating pain. Once the problematic muscles are identified, Marcus injects the muscle attachments and the belly of the muscle. While he uses lidocaine, for the patient's comfort, the mechanism of action is the needle itself. Marcus reported that his method deviates from the standard of care, which is to palpate muscles to identify which muscles have trigger points. This often leads to identification of the wrong muscle for injection, according to Marcus; consequently, the improvements are short-lived. The standard of care furthermore involves injecting the trigger point itself, which Marcus has found is not as effective as injecting the muscle attachments and belly. Marcus's injections are followed by physical therapy. Also, his patients are instructed in a home exercise program based on the Kraus-Weber exercises, which are discussed in chapter 9.

Myofascial pain is poorly understood by treating physicians, who usually fail to understand that trigger points are not the only possible muscle-pain generators, according to Marcus in a 2010 article. Muscle weakness, stiffness, spasm, or tension can also cause pain and need to be evaluated and treated for successful pain resolution. In the article, Marcus reported on 45 patients he identified as having "muscle pain amenable to injection" (MPAI) and treated according to the treatment protocol he had developed. A group of patients who met the MPAI criteria but were not yet treated served as the control group. One month after treatment, pain had decreased an average of 62%, pain interference with daily activities decreased 68%, and treated patients were doing significantly better than the control group.[9]

In a subsequent study (2013), 56 patients who had all failed an invasive treatment—back surgery, epidural steroid injections, facet blocks, or trigger point injection—were treated using Marcus's protocol. At a median follow-up of 77 weeks, pain severity had dropped significantly, with 52% of the respondents reporting over 50% relief. Three of seven patients originally scheduled for spine surgery canceled their surgeries and reported significant relief at follow-up.[10]

Marcus refers his patients to other kinds of therapies when indicated, including psychological therapies, massage, and interdisciplinary pain programs. Since there are no interdisciplinary pain programs left in New York City, Marcus refers his patients to the Johns Hopkins Pain Treatment Center in Baltimore, Maryland, or the Pain Management Center at the University of Miami.[11]

The comprehensive nature of Marcus's interventions, in which he not only treats all aspects of the muscle problem but also evaluates the whole person and refers for other therapies as needed, probably contributes significantly to the superior outcomes he achieves with his injection therapy, compared to other types of injection therapies.

Mary

I was able to interview several patients who had complex pain conditions and were significantly helped by Marcus, including 28-year-old Mary, who was diagnosed with fibromyalgia at age 11. Fibromyalgia is a chronic pain condition characterized by the presence of at least 11 "tender points" that cause widespread pain.[12]

Mary's condition might have started with a tennis injury. Her doctor started her on antidepressants, but her pain grew progressively worse. Her daily pain levels were 6 to 7 on a 10-point scale, with flare-ups that raised her pain level to a 10. Though offered opioids, she didn't want to be sedated. She tried nutritional approaches, including a protein and vegetable diet and then a vegetarian diet and finally 60 to 70 supplements. None of it helped. She was intermittently home-schooled during her flare-ups.

Despite her difficulties, Mary decided to attend college. At that point, she elected to use a low dose of Vicodin to help her cope. She sometimes used a wheelchair to get around, particularly when traveling. She tried some other antidepressants. She also took a vitamin cocktail IV weekly, which helped with energy, which in turn helped her move, which in turn helped ease her pain a little. Her daily pain level was a 7 to 8 at this point.

Mary (cont.)

Mary persisted and attended graduate school, for social work, while continuing to try to manage her pain. She saw osteopaths, chiropractors, and acupuncturists and had PT on and off, as well as psychotherapy that included cognitive behavioral therapy and mindfulness training. Those therapies helped a little, but Mary did not begin getting any significant relief until she saw Marcus.

Marcus identified 100 muscles in need of treatment. Over a period of a year and a half, all of the identified muscles were injected, some more than once.

Since Mary completed her intensive treatment with Marcus about a year and a half ago, her daily pain levels have become a more manageable 3. She still sometimes has flare-ups, but they are less frequent and don't last as long. She occasionally uses opioids—but a lot less than before.

Gail

Gail, 33 years old, started having chronic pain at the age of 25. An elite rower who practiced with her team five hours a day, she hurt her shoulder rowing, and then her hip. She next sustained a back injury. For what was diagnosed as torn cartilage, she underwent two surgeries on her hip, which cost $60,000 each. The pain, however, didn't change. Her surgeon eventually apologized to her because the surgery had been unnecessary. Gail also had a series of pain injections. She was still in a great deal of pain but was wary of using opioids: her family had a history of drug and alcohol problems. Her younger brother died of an accidental overdose of muscle relaxants and sedatives at 23, shortly after Gail's pain problems started. Gail tried to manage her pain with Advil and Tylenol, but she ended up with an ulcer.

Gail (cont.)

Her daily pain levels were a 5 to 6 but sometimes flared up to an 8 to 10. Sometimes, she almost passed out from the pain. At one point, Gail, a physical therapist, was out of work for six months. Psychotherapy, acupuncture, and massage kept her able to function at her work, but she was miserable from the pain.

Then one day Gail came across Marcus's book and decided to contact him. He spent more than 45 minutes on the phone with her explaining the treatment and answering her questions. After the injections, her pain immediately decreased. Gail compared the treatment to peeling the layers of an onion. Sometimes the injections were at sites that were not anywhere near the pain.

At 18 months since her treatment with Marcus, Gail reports she is no longer in chronic pain and can walk for several hours. The only discomfort she experiences now is the normal muscle pain that follows activity. Her insurance carrier initially refused to pay for the treatment, which cost somewhere between $5,000 and $8,000, but eventually agreed to pay.

Thomas

Dr. Thomas Blanck is a colleague of Dr. Marcus at NYU Medical School, where he is a professor in the Department of Anesthesiology. In 1999, Thomas herniated a disc while stretching, which led to pain and paralysis in his left leg. Disc surgery alleviated the pain and weakness, but he later herniated the disc again, this time undergoing a spinal fusion. Since then, he has experienced intermittent back and leg pain that interferes with normal activities.

Thomas (cont.)

At 70 years old, Thomas still likes to stay active by, among other activities, playing tennis. When his pain flared up in the past, he would go to physical therapy, which helped but took a long time. Now he sees Marcus for flare-ups and finds he can get back to his usual activities more quickly, though he does report he still has trouble sitting for long periods of time. Marcus treats him with injections or laser therapy.

Thomas also reports that his son was successfully treated by Marcus. His son, who had severe upper back and shoulder pain from swimming injuries, had been subjected to many surgeries before meeting Marcus. Marcus was able to help him decrease pain and improve range of motion with injection treatments.

Chapter 4

Surgical Treatments

A common intervention for many types of pain, surgery is often used to treat back pain, especially low-back pain, along with neck and knee pain, particularly pain caused by osteoarthritis. Surgical treatments for pain have met with varying success. And complications from surgery can be worse than the original disorder.

Spinal Surgery for Back Pain

The number of spinal surgeries has been steadily increasing in recent decades. In one five-year period alone, from 1997 to 2002, the annual number of spinal surgeries more than tripled, from 317,000 to more than 1 million.[1] Even before these increases, back surgery rates were two to five times higher in the United States than in other industrialized nations.[2]

A 1999 study found wide disparity in the number of spinal surgeries in different regions across Maine. It also found that the best surgical outcomes, in terms of improvement in pain levels and function, occurred in areas with the lowest surgical rates.[3] Some experts have suggested that reducing the number of unnecessary surgeries would produce a reduction in surgical complication greater than that from improving the technical quality of surgical procedures.[4]

Failed back surgery syndrome (FBSS) is a term used to describe the persistence or recurrence of low-back pain after spinal surgery. Research has shown that the more surgeries a patient has, the less likely an operation is to successfully relieve pain. In one study, the success rate for initial surgeries was over 50%; success of second surgeries was 30%; third surgeries 15%; and fourth surgeries 5%.[5]

Different kinds of spinal surgery have differing success rates, with the worst success rate in spinal fusion. One review found that the failure rate of lumbar fusion surgery was between 30% and 46%; disc surgery, 19% and 25%; and decompression surgery for spinal stenosis, 35% and 36%.[6] Another review noted that, despite advances in surgical technology, there has been no decline in the rate of failed back surgery.[7] According to two randomized controlled trials of disc surgery, the short-term outcome for surgery was superior to nonsurgical management; however, two years later the nonsurgical group had outcomes similar to those of the surgical group.[8,9] Authors of a 2002 systematic review of disc-replacement surgery were unable to find reports of any controlled trials. They found the evidence on effectiveness so sparse and the complication rates so high that they recommended that total disc replacements be considered experimental procedures used only in "strict clinical trials."[10]

Not only may surgery fail to help but it can also worsen the patient's condition by creating spinal instability or misalignment, injuring nerve roots, or tearing the covering of the spinal cord, or because of wound infection.[11]

A 1997 study found the estimated annual cost of medical therapy for patients with FBSS, excluding costs for further surgery or surgically implanted devices, was $18,883 per patient in the United States.[12]

Studies have shown that psychological factors predict disability due to low-back pain better than structural abnormalities.[13] Patients with significant levels of anxiety or depression or who have poor coping skills or somatization (conversion of emotional distress into physical symptoms) have poor outcomes for spinal surgery.[14,15] An association has also been seen between the presence of a workers' compensation claim and poor surgical outcome.[16,17,18,19] The latter may be due to the extreme stress associated with being on workers' compensation, as noted in chapter 5, more than a desire to not work and to collect benefits.

A 1992 study of 86 patients who had lumbar spine surgery found a highly significant correlation between unsuccessful surgery and a history of childhood trauma. The more types of childhood trauma experienced, the higher the rate of unsuccessful surgery. Patients in the study had psychiatric evaluations to determine the presence or absence of five types of childhood trauma: physical abuse, sexual abuse, alcohol or drug abuse by a primary caregiver, abandonment, and emotional neglect or abuse. Patients with no childhood trauma had a surgical success rate of 95%. Patients with one type of childhood trauma had a success rate of 75%. With two types of trauma, patients' surgical success rate declined to 43%. Those with three types of childhood trauma had a 20% success rate; with four types, 7%; and with five, 0%. The authors recommended a preoperative psychological review, and suggested that if three or more psychological factors are present, surgery should be avoided "unless there is overwhelming spinal pathology."[20]

A study published in 1998 found that experienced British spinal surgeons subjectively identified psychologically distressed patients only 26% of the time.[21] A study published in 2000 evaluated how well a presurgical screening instrument could predict whether a spinal surgery would be successful. Presurgical psychological screening (PPS) was performed on 204 spinal surgery patients to evaluate the presence of psychological and medical risk factors for each patient, and a surgical prognosis of good, fair, or poor was determined. The PPS predicted poor surgical outcome with 82% accuracy. Of 53 patients predicted to have a poor outcome, only 9 achieved fair or good results from their surgery.[22] Despite all the evidence of the importance of psychological factors in surgical success, a 2012 U.S. study found that only 37% of surgeons responding to a survey used presurgical psychological screening. Use was highest among those in practice more than 14 years and those who performed more than 200 surgeries annually.[23]

Another Questionable Procedure

There have been numerous reports of questionable surgical implants in recent years. Implants used in spinal surgery are no exception. The US Senate Finance Committee recently investigated whether Medtronic had improperly influenced studies of its bone-growth product InFuse, which is used in spinal fusion surgery. The investigation found that over a period of four years, Medtronic had paid approximately $210 million to physician-authors who were heavily involved in writing medical journal articles, and that these financial ties were not disclosed to the medical journals. As a result of these conflicts of interest, the journal articles did not include a complete list of adverse events associated with InFuse and overstated the problems associated with an alternative technique that used the patient's own bone.

Testimony by an independent physician to an FDA advisory panel before the approval of InFuse was written by Medtronics, and the physician, Dr. Hal Mathew, was later hired as a vice president of Medtronics.[24] FDA approval was limited to one specific type of spinal fusion surgery, but off-label (nonapproved) use has been found to account for 85% of sales.[25] In 2008, the FDA issued a public health warning that the off-label use of InFuse in surgery in the cervical spine (neck area) was associated with life-threatening swelling in patients' throats and necks.[26] A few years later, the FDA refused to approve a higher-strength version of InFuse, called Amplify, out of concern that it might cause cancer. The possible connection of Amplify to cancer was not reported in the industry-sponsored studies.[27] One physician researcher and critic, Dr. Eugene Carragee of Stanford University, reported that many doctors were using InFuse at levels near or exceeding the Amplify dosage. [28]

MRIs Don't Accurately Identify the Source of Back Pain

The relationship between spinal abnormalities, often targeted with surgery, and low-back pain has long been controversial. Over a period of more than 20 years, between 1984 and 2005, many MRI and CT scan studies were conducted on asymptomatic people from all walks of life. All of these studies found a large percentage of people with disc bulges or protrusions (contained herniations) or degenerated discs who had no back pain. For instance, a 1990 MRI study of asymptomatic adults found that of those younger than 60, 22% had herniated discs, 54% had bulging discs, and 46% had a degenerative disc. The same study found that among asymptomatic adults older than 60, 36% had a herniated disc, 79% had a bulging disc, and 93% had a degenerative disc.[29] A 1994 study evaluated the frequency of abnormal MRI scans of the lumbar (lower) spine in people without back pain. Only 36% of the 98 asymptomatic participants had normal discs at all levels. The older the individual, the more likely she was to have structural abnormalities of the spine. The authors of the study concluded that given the high prevalence of abnormal findings in asymptomatic individuals and the high prevalence of back pain, the discovery of disc abnormalities in people with back pain may frequently be coincidental, and have nothing to do with their back pain.[30] Finding that more than 90% of lower-spine MRIs in adults are abnormal, authors of a 1997 review of MRIs for back pain came to similar conclusions.[31]

The hypothesis that those with abnormal findings would soon develop back pain was disproved in a 2001 study that followed studied individuals for seven years. The findings on the initial MRIs did not predict the development or duration of low-back pain.[32]

Cheron

A particularly egregious story about the misuse of an MRI in the diagnosis and treatment of chronic pain was reported in a 2014 *Washington Post* article. Cheron Wicker developed chronic, excruciating pain in the tip of her index finger. In the course of consulting many specialists over a seven-year period, Wicker was given an MRI that showed herniated discs in her neck. The physician concluded that the cause of her index finger pain was a pinched nerve caused by the herniated discs. After spinal surgery to replace two herniated discs failed to have any impact on the problem, Cheron was persuaded to undergo a second spinal surgery to address another herniated disc in her neck. Again, she experienced no relief. Medication, including narcotics, also had no impact on the pain. The pain was so bad that at one point Cheron considered self-amputation of her finger. Finally a hand surgeon discovered the actual cause of her pain: a small, rare benign glomus tumor under her fingernail. When the fingernail and tumor were removed, Cheron finally had relief from her pain.[33]

Another diagnostic tool for determining whether a disc is responsible for chronic back pain and surgery is indicated, provocative discography is generally used after positive MRI findings. The procedure involves injecting a contrast dye into the disc space to obtain more information on disc structure and to determine whether the injection provokes pain similar to that usually experienced by the patient. If similar pain is provoked, the patient is considered a candidate for spinal fusion surgery.

Patients who had positive findings on provocative discography and elected to have spinal surgery were compared to those who opted for more conservative treatment—including physical therapy, epidural injections, and medications—in a study published in 2014. At long-term follow-up of an average of five years, both groups had improved, but there was no significant difference between the two groups regarding pain, general health status, or disability.[34]

When Back Surgery Might Be Necessary

Surgery should be considered when a herniated disc squeezes a nerve in the back that causes pain from the buttock to the toes and there is numbness, weakness, muscle shrinkage, and reduced reflexes, along with loss of control of urination and defecation. Similarly, surgery should be considered when a herniated disc presses upon a nerve in the neck and causes numbness, weakness, reduced reflexes, and muscle shrinkage in the arms and hands.[35]

Even when some of these signs and symptoms are present, surgery may not relieve the pain if the herniated disc is not the true source of the problem.[36]

Another instance in which surgery might be considered for back pain is when the spine is unstable because of slippage of the vertebrae, a condition known as spondylolisthesis. Too much movement of the vertebrae back and forth can cause pain. Small amounts of movement back and forth may not be the real cause of the pain, and spinal fusion, the recommended procedure for this problem, may cause more problems later on because of the stress a partially immobilized spine puts on other parts of the spine.[37]

Knee Surgery

Surgical treatment is also often recommended for painful knees. Arthroscopic knee surgery for osteoarthritis provides a blatant example of how an untested surgical procedure can achieve—and maintain—widespread use, despite growing evidence of its ineffectiveness.

In a study published in 2002 in the *New England Journal of Medicine,* 180 patients with osteoarthritis of the knee were randomly assigned to receive arthroscopic surgery or placebo surgery. In arthroscopic surgery, a small incision is made in the knee to remove cartilage fragments and smooth the joint surfaces. Patients in the placebo group received a simulated procedure. Patients were assessed at multiple points over a 24-month period with the use of self-reported scores for pain and function along with one objective test of walking and stair climbing. At no point did the intervention group report less pain or better function than the placebo group.[38] Physicians as well as insurers largely ignored this study.

In another study published in the *New England Journal of Medicine* in 2008, it was reported that physical therapy and painkillers were just as effective at reducing pain and improving mobility as arthroscopic knee surgery for osteoarthritis.[39] In the study, 178 adults were given physical therapy and painkillers such as ibuprofen. Around half also underwent arthroscopic orthopedic surgery. At various stages afterward, both groups reported similar improvements in joint pain, stiffness, and mobility. The surgery provided no extra benefit.[40]

Another widely used surgery for knee pain is arthroscopic surgery for degenerative meniscal tears. A meta-analysis published in 2014 in the *Canadian Medical Association Journal* of seven randomized controlled trials of surgery for meniscal tears in middle-aged people found that the surgery provided no benefit for improving either function or pain compared to management without surgery.[41] Younger athletes with meniscal tears from athletic injuries may benefit from surgery to repair the knee.[42]

Summary: Pharmaceutical and Surgical Treatments for Pain

Surgical and pharmaceutical treatments for pain are often costly, dangerous, and ineffective, with most pain patients continuing to suffer tremendously. Some are worse off as a result of their treatments. Their suffering and impaired productivity significantly impacts their families and communities, along with our national economy.

A study published in the *Journal of the American Medical Association* in 2013, "Worsening Trends in the Management and Treatment of Back Pain," found that from 1999 to 2010, despite the publication of numerous clinical guidelines recommending conservative treatment of back and neck pain, there had been a large and statistically significant increase in the use of narcotics, MRIs, CT scans, and referrals for invasive medical procedures.[43]

CHAPTER 5
MIND/BODY TREATMENTS

Mind/body treatments for chronic pain include psychotherapy, including cognitive behavioral therapy (CBT) and trauma resolution techniques; relaxation training; biofeedback; meditation; laughter therapy; hypnosis; and guided visualization. These types of treatment are among the most potent tools for effective pain management. They have the added benefit of being completely safe and low cost. Furthermore, most are available for self-care.

The underlying physiology of the mind/body connection in chronic pain is now well known. The brain is an active component in pain, interpreting nerve signals from the body and then creating the experience of pain. This process is important for survival—we can be alerted to danger and avoid it. However, when we react to pain with fear, anger, anxiety, or frustration, our responses tend to reinforce pain pathways and increase pain. Life stressors—including those that result from being in pain—such as loss of income, more difficult relationships, and childhood trauma, also result in increased pain.[1]

Stress and Pain

For most people, chronic pain is not a result of pathological tissue changes but rather physiological changes precipitated by chronic stress cause pain. When our minds perceive a threat, this activates certain brain regions, which cause the autonomic nervous system to trigger the fight or-flight response. As a result, the body increases muscle tension, heart rate, and blood pressure and restricts blood flow to the peripheral tissues while suppressing digestion, immunity, and healing. The purpose of these physiological changes is to direct the most energy possible toward saving the person's life in the moment of danger. These physiological changes, if chronically triggered, can cause changes in nerve-firing patterns and brain-wiring patterns that cause chronic pain and many other disorders.[2]

Another connection between emotional stress and pain is breath—when people are stressed, their breathing is shallower. This deprives the muscles of the oxygen they need for normal functioning and can create or exacerbate pain.[3]

Low-back pain, neck pain, jaw pain, and tension headaches can all occur as a result of muscle tension. Functional magnetic resonance imaging (fMRI) studies have shown that when pain patients have negative thoughts, areas of the brain associated with pain perception are activated and pain sensations intensify.[4]

Emotional responses increase the activity of a part of the brain called the anterior cingulate cortex (ACC). When the ACC is more active, pain increases.[5,6] In addition, when the ACC is activated, the dorsolateral prefrontal cortex (DLPFC), which decreases pain signals, is turned off.[7]

Many studies have shown the connection between emotions and physiological responses that cause pain. For example, anger can cause unconscious increases in tension in the back muscles of people in chronic pain. This muscle tension can create severe pain.[8] Also, suppressing anger has been shown to increase pain perception[9] and physiological reactivity.[10] People who have experienced childhood trauma are much more likely to develop chronic pain as adults than those who have not experienced such trauma because their autonomic nervous systems are chronically more activated.[11]

Psychologists Peter Levine and Maggie Phillips, coauthors of *Freedom from Pain*, believe that unresolved trauma, held in the body, causes chronic pain for many people. They report that during their 80 combined years of clinical experience, they have discovered that pain that did not respond to any of the usual treatments could be traced back to unprocessed accumulated stress and trauma. Unresolved trauma from childhood—such as illness, hospitalizations, surgeries, birth trauma, attachment trauma, and physical and emotional neglect and abuse—can all get stirred up by a current event, including the onset of pain. Levine and Phillips found that most people in unrelenting pain were not taught early in life how to deal effectively with uncomfortable or distressing experiences, either because of neglect or because they were abused when they expressed distress. The way out of pain for these individuals, say Levine and Phillips, is to learn how to calm themselves in the aftermath of disturbing experiences.[12]

Conditioned responses can also play a role in chronic pain. Any stimulus present at the time a pain episode occurs—a food, a person, an activity—can become associated with pain and trigger another pain episode upon re-exposure.[13]

Relief from Pain with Mind/Body Interventions

Physiological changes that create pain are reversible with mind/body interventions that decrease activation, increase relaxation, or appropriately discharge or process emotions.

Mind/body interventions can also increase the body's own ability to treat pain. The body produces natural painkillers, known as endorphins. Endorphins are one of a class of brain chemicals known as neurotransmitters and are found throughout the brain and nervous system. Beyond providing pain relief, the release of endorphins leads to enhancement of the immune response and feelings of euphoria. Mental activities that increase release of endorphins include laughing,[14] thinking about pleasurable activities, and meditation.[15] Physical exercise also increases endorphin release, an effect commonly known as "runner's high."[16] Endorphins bind to receptors on cells throughout the body to produce their effect. It is these natural receptors that prescription opioids bind to in order to decrease pain.[17] Chronic use of prescription opioids reduces the body's production of endorphins.[18] Unlike prescription opioids, high-endorphin production by the body is not associated with addiction, dependence, or overdose.

Thousands of studies have demonstrated the effectiveness of mind/body treatments in alleviating chronic pain. An exhaustive review of the literature is beyond the scope of this book; however, some of the most effective mind/body treatments will be described and a few studies of each will be reviewed.

Cognitive Behavioral Therapy

Cognitive behavioral therapy (CBT) is based on the idea that thoughts affect behavior and emotions and that changing maladaptive thoughts can improve mood and functioning. Many chronic pain patients fear the consequences of their pain and worry about their ability to cope with it. They may have unrealistic fears that their resumption of normal activities at home and at work will result in further injury. These thoughts and fears may prolong or prevent recovery. CBT uses cognitive restructuring (replacing unhelpful beliefs with more positive ones) and behavioral experiments, such as gradual exposure to feared situations and activities, to improve emotional and physical well-being.

A 2012 meta-analysis of 46 randomized controlled studies of CBT for chronic low-back pain found that when compared with wait-list controls, CBT had the following effects:

Reduced

- Pain
- Anxiety
- Avoidance
- Back-related worry
- Catastrophizing
- Depression
- Disability
- Stress

Increased

- Coping
- Health-related quality of life (females
- only)
- Pain control
- Pain self-efficacy
- Perceived ability to function
- General quality of life
- Social support

CBT also offers economic benefits in terms of reduced health care visits, reduction in work days lost, and higher likelihood of return of work.[19]

Many studies have shown that CBT and exercise in combination were as effective as back surgery over both the short and long term, with lower costs and fewer risks.[20,21,22,23,24,25]

Relaxation Training

It makes intuitive sense, based on what is now known about the connection between chronic pain and stress, that learning to become more relaxed would result in reduced pain. There are two types of relaxation techniques: active and passive. Active, or progressive, relaxation, produces lower arousal as specific muscles are voluntarily tensed and relaxed, and as the individual learns to differentiate between relaxation and tension. Passive relaxation includes deep breathing or using words or imagery to induce lower arousal. Meditation, for instance, involves focusing on a calming or neutral word or phrase to the exclusion of everything else, including habitual worries or fears. When negative stimuli are removed, the body moves toward relaxation. Effective relaxation strategies involve practicing the techniques frequently until a relaxed state can be achieved quickly in any time of need. This level of training in relaxation is called training to mastery.

Results of studies on relaxation as a treatment for chronic pain have found that different behavioral interventions that have a relaxing effect tend to significantly reduce pain, though there is not enough evidence to determine which relaxation techniques are most effective for which disorders. No studies have reported any negative side effects of relaxation training.[26]

A multidisciplinary technology assessment panel convened by the National Institutes of Health in 1996 to evaluate the evidence base for behavioral and relaxation approaches in the treatment of chronic pain and insomnia found that the evidence was strong for the use of relaxation techniques in alleviating chronic pain in many medical conditions.[27]

A 2012 Cochrane review of studies found that, for children and adolescents, there was good evidence that relaxation is effective in reducing the frequency and severity of chronic pain in chronic headache, recurrent abdominal pain, fibromyalgia, sickle cell disease, and juvenile arthritis, and that relaxation reduces disability for many chronic pain conditions in children.

Biofeedback

Biofeedback uses sensitive electronic instruments to measure a person's bodily processes and then feeds back that information to the person so that control of the physiology can be learned. Several types of biofeedback—including muscle tension (EMG), temperature (blood flow), heart rate variability (HRV), and brain wave (neurofeedback)—have been shown to be helpful for reducing chronic pain. Biofeedback is often paired with coaching in relaxation techniques.

Biofeedback can enhance the effectiveness of relaxation training by giving the patient information on the effectiveness of his efforts. Biofeedback takes measurements on the surface of the body, and this information is used as part of an educational process. It is completely safe and without negative side effects.

A 2008 review found that biofeedback treatment was effective for the following chronic pain conditions:

- Low-back pain
- Neck pain
- Abdominal pain
- Jaw pain
- Phantom limb pain
- Fibromyalgia
- Complex regional pain syndrome
- Migraine and tension headaches[28]

In a 1993 study comparing EMG biofeedback, cognitive behavioral therapy, and conservative medical management for back pain and temporomandibular joint (jaw) pain, the biofeedback group had the most positive changes posttreatment. At 6- and 24-month follow-ups, only the biofeedback group had maintained significant improvements in pain severity, interference with daily activities, emotional distress, and reductions in use of the health care system for pain treatment.[29] In another study, 50 chronic pain patients were randomly assigned to a biofeedback-plus-relaxation training group or a pain education group. The biofeedback/relaxation group reported significantly less pain and anxiety compared to the pain education group.[30] A study of recurrent abdominal pain in 64 children and teenagers using thermal biofeedback alone or in combination with cognitive behavioral therapy found that pain was significantly improved compared to an inactive (fiber-only) treatment control group.[31]

A study on migraines found superior results for biofeedback-assisted relaxation compared to self-directed relaxation.[32] Another study found that six sessions of EMG biofeedback treatment resulted in a significant drop in chronic tension headaches, compared to the complete lack of improvement in a control group.[33] A review of migraine treatments published by the American Academy of Neurology in 2000 concluded that temperature and muscle biofeedback with relaxation training were effective and recommended biofeedback as a treatment option.[34]

My Story

The skills learned in a short episode of biofeedback treatment are available for a lifetime of self-managed care. My own introduction to alternative medicine began with biofeedback. In 1977, when I was 25 years old, I injured my back after taking up running to get in better shape. I went to a doctor at my HMO who told me to stop running. And even though I did, things continued to get worse. Everything that I did to try to heal myself, including back exercises, injured my back more. After a few months, I was in so much pain that I could no longer function and had to drop out of graduate school, where I was studying for a master's degree in social work. For the next three years, I could barely function, and I was in constant agony as I went from doctor to doctor.

The doctors prescribed medications that left me feeling like a zombie while doing nothing for the pain. Some of the medications were very dangerous. I learned that one of them could cause leukemia after only two weeks of administration.

My HMO refused to pay for a chiropractor, so I paid out of pocket. The chiropractor validated that my pain wasn't all in my head. Using a heat-sensing instrument, he could pinpoint on any given day the area of my back with the most pain by measuring the heat from the inflammation. Chiropractic treatment lowered my pain levels a little, but I was still in too much pain to function. I was thinking about suicide.

Then my friend Vicki Zeldin, a health reporter for a local newspaper, suggested I read *Anatomy of an Illness* by Norman Cousins. Cousins had laughed his way to better health after being diagnosed with a painful, progressively crippling joint disease. Cousins wrote extensively about the mind/body connection and mentioned biofeedback.

My Story (cont.)

I found a psychologist in my area, Dr. Martin Leyden, who offered biofeedback treatment. In my first session, Leyden explained to me that worrying about the pain caused more tension and more pain. He instructed me in simple techniques to clear my mind and reduce stress while he measured my success with hand temperature biofeedback. (Cold hands are indicators of stress.) Leyden provided me with a $5 biofeedback device that I could wrap around my finger to measure my hand temperature so that I could practice at home. After the first session with the psychologist, my pain levels diminished about 50%. I now knew that I had a way of managing my pain. Instead of worrying about my pain level, I could turn my attention to lowering it. After two or three sessions, all that I could afford, I was on my own. I monitored my hand temperature and worked on relaxing and warming my hands throughout the day. The more I practiced, the better I felt.

Gradually, using biofeedback and other mind/body techniques, I was able to get back to work, finish my master's degree, and become a fully functioning human being and contributing member of society again. I credit biofeedback with not only healing my pain but also saving my life. In the 35 years since I was treated, I have never taken even a single dose of a prescription painkiller and have very rarely taken even an over-the-counter one. In addition, biofeedback gave me a completely different outlook on how to manage my health. I have used that perspective ever since to stay healthy and to address other health challenges that have come up.

Twenty-two years ago I became a certified biofeedback practitioner and have successfully used biofeedback to help many others with chronic pain and other medical conditions.

Jane

The advantages in pain relief of biofeedback over relaxation training alone are illustrated by one of my clients, whom I'll call Jane. Ever since a serious car accident, Jane had suffered from severe neck and back pain. As part of her attempts to resolve the pain, she was meditating three hours a day. After hearing this, I wondered what I could do to help her, as she was already doing a great deal of relaxation practice. I conducted a biofeedback session with her during which I monitored muscle tension in her shoulder (upper trapezius) muscles while she engaged in her usual meditation practice. I found that the longer she meditated, the more tense her shoulders became. Muscle tension increases pain. I brought her attention to this and had her practice the meditation with biofeedback. She learned to be more aware of her muscle tension and how to control it, and her pain level decreased significantly.

Susan

One of my colleagues, Susan Antelis, a licensed mental health counselor and board-certified biofeedback practitioner on Long Island, experienced dramatic healing results from biofeedback that inspired her career direction. Susan had started having hormonally triggered classic migraines with aura monthly when she was 13. Migraine headaches had occurred in her family for generations, and Susan's would last for days at a time. At that time, in 1966, medication was not used in children. Susan's headaches worsened to the point that she was experiencing them three days a week. Her father was a doctor, and his partner told Susan that she'd have the headaches for the rest of her life.

Susan (cont.)

The headaches were so bad that Susan didn't know if she'd be able to finish high school or go to college. At age 19, Susan consulted another doctor, who put her on medication for headaches. The medication left her wired and hung over for three days after a headache. By age 20, Susan was very depressed and almost suicidal. That's when she decided to find a therapist.

Psychologist Glenda Axel was up on new ways and referred Susan to Gretchen Randolph for biofeedback. Susan was treated weekly with hand temperature biofeedback and EMG (muscle) biofeedback. Though she found it frustrating at first, after 10 months, Susan was almost headache free. She continued to carry her medication around with her for three years, but she never used it again. In 1980, Susan took her first professional biofeedback training course and bought her own equipment. Her migraines stopped completely in 1981. Susan started training her own two daughters in biofeedback when they were three years old. When they were 13, they started having migraines but were able to stop them with biofeedback.

More recently, neurofeedback (brain wave biofeedback) has been shown helpful for some extremely challenging pain conditions. A 2006 study found significant differences in the brain electrical activity (EEGs) of fibromyalgia sufferers compared to age- and gender-matched healthy participants.[35] Other studies have also shown abnormalities in the EEGs of chronic pain patients with other types of pain.[36,37,38] These abnormalities, which included overactivation in many brain regions, can be ameliorated with neurofeedback, resulting in a decrease in pain.

A randomized controlled study in 2010 found that those with fibromyalgia who were treated with 20 sessions of neurofeedback over a four-week period showed significant improvements in pain and fatigue levels, both during treatment and at 24-month follow-up. These improvements were much greater than those achieved by the other study group, which used an SSRI antidepressant for treatment.[39]

Quantitative EEG, or QEEG, is a brain mapping technique that identifies abnormalities in brain regions and brain connections, which can then be corrected with neurofeedback. In 2011, a migraine headache study compared QEEG-guided neurofeedback to pharmaceutical treatment. Fifty-four percent of patients in the neurofeedback group experienced a complete remission of migraine headaches. An additional 39% experienced a decrease in migraine frequency of greater than 50%. In contrast, of patients in the study who elected to continue on drug therapy, 68% experienced no change in headache frequency, and only 8% achieved a reduction of greater than 50%.[40]

A 2013 study found that neurofeedback reduced pain in spinal cord injury patients, both during the 12-session treatment period and at the three-month follow-up.[41]

None of the biofeedback or neurofeedback studies reported any negative side effects. In fact, it is common to see improvements in other health conditions and general well-being as a result of biofeedback treatment.

Unfortunately, you will most likely be on your own when it comes to accessing biofeedback or neurofeedback treatments for chronic pain or any other condition. Most insurance companies refuse to pay for biofeedback treatment, and few physicians will tell you about it.

Another problem with access to biofeedback treatment is that there are very few biofeedback practitioners. Biofeedback providers are usually health care professionals licensed in psychology, social work, nursing, medicine, or other health care specialties. Becoming a biofeedback practitioner requires extensive additional training beyond the health care license as well as purchase of specialized equipment. Since insurance reimbursement is either unavailable or, in those rare cases when it is available, reimbursed at rates lower than those for other medical interventions, health care providers are discouraged from offering biofeedback treatment.

Emotional Awareness and Processing

Can you cure chronic pain just by paying more attention to your feelings? Yes, according to Dr. John Sarno, who coined the term *tension myositis syndrome* (TMS), and Dr. Howard Schubiner, who coined the term *mindbody syndrome* (MBS) to describe the pain and other illness caused by suppressed emotions. Another term used to refer to the syndrome is *psychophysiologic disorder* (PPD).[42] Schubiner reported that people who have had significant childhood trauma and those who have personality traits of guilt, self-criticism, low self-esteem, high expectations for self, extreme responsibility for others, and self-sacrifice are most likely to develop MBS. Powerlessness, whether real or perceived, also can trigger MBS. Often the emotions or situations causing MBS are so unacceptable or shameful to the person that her unconscious mind keeps them hidden from consciousness. Feelings that we are unaware of are most likely to cause physical symptoms, including pain.[43]

Sarno, the author of *Healing Back Pain*[44] and *The Mindbody Prescription*, claims an almost 100% recovery rate with an intervention that consists solely of educating patients about the repressed emotion/chronic pain connection.[45] In an investigative report in July 1999 by ABC TV newsmagazine *20/20,* 20 random patient files were pulled from Sarno's records and these patients were then contacted. Three additional patients were followed in real time. Many of the patients had tried all available conventional and alternative treatments without relief of their pain. After being treated by Sarno, all 23 patients had rapid and dramatic improvements in their pain symptoms and were able to maintain that improvement over time. One of the reporters in the *20/20* segment had himself been treated by Sarno, many years earlier, and had experienced dramatic lasting improvements in his back pain. This reporter was unable to convince his brother, who suffered from similar back issues and was a physician, to even consider Sarno's approach. His brother continued to suffer.[46]

Schubiner's program, described in his book *Unlearn Your Pain*, builds on Sarno's approach. He reported that it works by activating the conscious part of the brain to override the subconscious pathways creating MBS. It begins with a simple statement: "I have MBS and I can cure myself."

According to Schubiner, feelings of fear, anger, resentment, guilt, shame, sadness, and grief need to be experienced, expressed, and released in order to heal mindbody syndrome. His program guides pain sufferers through a process to do this. Verbal expression and expressive writing are part of the process.[47] When symptoms arise, including pain, patients are instructed to remind themselves there is nothing wrong with their body and that the symptoms are just a way of warning them about the presence of negative feelings.[48]

Research Results

In a study of fibromyalgia patients using Schubiner's emotion processing approach, six weeks after treatment, 25% of patients were in remission while another 25% had experienced a moderate improvement in their pain levels. These improvements were still present after six months. In contrast, none of the patients in the usual care control group showed any improvement in pain levels.[49]

Psychologist James Pennebaker has made studying the physiological effects of emotional inhibition and emotional expression his life's work. In his 1997 book *Opening Up: The Healing Power of Expressing Emotions,* Pennebaker reported that emotional inhibition is hard physical work—we must exert effort not to think, feel, or act. The effort involved in inhibition takes its toll on our health over time, resulting in many physical problems, including chronic pain. Actively confronting negative experiences by acknowledging our feelings and thinking, writing, and talking about our experiences reduces the strain on the body caused by inhibition. In addition, actively processing traumatic events in these ways allows us to come to a better understanding of negative experiences and allows us to move beyond them.[50] Once we see the connection between our pain and psychological issues, we can focus our energy on reducing the real cause of our distress. Understanding this cause-effect relationship also gives us a sense of control over our health, which further reduces our stress.[51]

Trauma Release Techniques

Other mind/body approaches to treating chronic pain focus on resolving past trauma. One such approach is somatic experiencing, developed by psychologist Peter Levine. Levine identified three types of pain: physical, caused by actual tissue damage; emotional, related to unresolved emotions stored in the body instead of being expressed; and posttraumatic, caused by reactions to overwhelming, terrifying, or devastating events.[52]

A traumatic event is one in which a person has been exposed to actual or perceived threats to his survival or physical wholeness that led to feelings of intense fear, helplessness, or loss of control. Trauma can involve a single incident or ongoing threats, such as childhood physical or emotional abuse. Generally speaking, the more trauma a person has experienced, the more likely he is to develop physical and emotional illnesses, including chronic pain.[53] Among injured people, those with PTSD experience more pain and respond less well to medical interventions than those who do not have the disorder.[54]

According to Levine, wild animals do not experience long-term trauma from stress because when they are threatened, if they survive, they complete the fight-or-flight response by either fighting back against what threatens them or fleeing the source of the threat. After the threat has passed, they literally shake off any residual effects of stress during a period of involuntary trembling.

In contrast, humans often can't escape or fight back, and we don't allow our bodies to shake off the residual energy from the threatening experience. We often shift into the freeze response, a state of helplessness and hopelessness that occurs when we believe there is no escape. This unprocessed energy is often at the root of pain.

Somatic Experiencing

The concept that traumatic stress is related to unprocessed energy from the trauma that exists in the nervous system and body, rather than the content of the event, is the foundation of somatic experiencing. It involves releasing the energy trapped in the nervous system by connecting with the body sensations related to the trauma and to our ability to adapt and recover so that healing can occur.[55]

EMDR

Another trauma resolution technique that has been successfully used for the treatment of chronic pain is eye movement desensitization and reprocessing (EMDR). In the late 1980s, Francine Shapiro, then a graduate student in psychology, was recalling an upsetting memory when her eyes spontaneously moved rapidly back and forth. Shapiro found she was significantly less distressed by the memory after this experience. Shapiro went on to experiment with the use of what has become known as bilateral stimulation/dual attention stimulus and discovered that the method could facilitate rapid resolution of PTSD, even in patients very resistant to treatment.[56] Subsequently, dozens of studies have shown positive results in the treatment of PTSD, which has led to widespread acceptance of EMDR for the treatment of this condition.

More recently there has been growing interest and research in the use of EMDR for chronic pain. EMDR has been shown to decrease physiological arousal and emotional distress as well as to increase relaxation and a feeling of distance from the problem, all of which have been found to reduce chronic pain.[57] When a traumatic memory includes chronic pain, resolving the traumatic memory is likely to help resolve the pain.[58] Even when pain is not caused by trauma, the physical discomfort and disability caused by severe, uncontrolled pain can be traumatizing in and of itself.[59]

Shapiro theorized that humans have a capacity for adaptive information processing (AIP). This refers to our capacity to learn from our experiences, which increases our ability to survive and thrive. Trauma overwhelms our nervous system's ability to process the memory, so that instead of learning from the experience, we store memories in fragments, we experience avoidance, and we never integrate the trauma. The EMDR process integrates the experience.[60] EMDR is an eight-step treatment process:

1. History taking
2. Assessment
3. Preparation
4. Desensitization
5. Installation
6. Body scan
7. Closure
8. Reevaluation

Many of these steps overlap with traditional psychotherapy. What makes EMDR unique is the desensitization and installation phases that include dual attention stimulus/bilateral stimulation. Clients are asked about their feelings and to rate the severity of distress on a scale of 0 to 10 (SUDs rating). They are then asked to identify a picture that represents the event, what they think about themselves in relation to the traumatic memory, how they would like to think about themselves in the future (positive cognition), and how true that positive statement seems to them at the moment on a scale of 1 to 7.[61]

During desensitization, clients are instructed to focus on the traumatic image, the negative self-statement, and associated feelings while also paying attention to a bilateral stimulation (finger movements, tapping, or sounds that move from side to side) for about 30 to 60 seconds (a set). Clients are directed to "just notice" and "let whatever happens happen." After each set, clients are instructed to take a deep breath and describe whatever feelings, sensations, thoughts, or memories they notice now. They are told to "just notice that," and then a new set is initiated. When clients report a SUDs of 0 or 1 while focusing on the memory, they are then instructed to focus on the previously identified positive cognition and to rate the strength of their belief in that statement. After EMDR processing, clients typically report that they feel more relaxed, less distressed by the memory, and better able to realistically evaluate current threats.[62]

The bilateral stimulation/dual attention component can also be used on its own as a pain management technique. This involves instructing the client to focus on her pain (including images and feelings) while simultaneously focusing on an audio tone or tapping bilateral stimulation and "letting whatever happens happen."[63]

Research Results

A 2014 review of all published studies on the use of EMDR in the treatment of chronic pain found 12 small studies, including 2 controlled and 10 observational. The studies were broken down as follows: 3 looked at the use of EMDR for phantom limb pain;[64,65,66] 2 evaluated migraine headaches;[67,68] 3 evaluated nonspecific musculoskeletal pain;[69,70,71] 2 assessed fibromyalgia;[72,73] and 1 had a mixed sample of chronic pain patients including those with headache, fibromyalgia, and neuropathic pain.[74] All studies found a significant reduction in pain intensity. Longer duration of treatment was associated with better results, and treatment effects were maintained or improved at follow-up (ranging from 3 months to 40 months). Those studies that also measured disability, depression, and anxiety additionally found improvements in those symptoms.[75] A study of EMDR in the treatment of nonspecific chronic back pain is currently underway, with published results expected in 2015.[76]

Energy Psychology Techniques

Another PTSD treatment that has been shown effective for chronic pain is emotional freedom technique (EFT). EFT is one of a group of interventions known as energy psychology. Energy psychology theory proposes that psychological problems are caused by disturbed patterns of energy in the mind/body communication system. As of 2014, more than 60 research studies had been published on energy psychology techniques, 59 showing significant positive results.[77]

Energy psychology techniques combine focused awareness on traumatic memories or physical or emotional distress with stimulation of the human energy field.[78] In EFT, acupuncture energy meridians are tapped at specific points while the client focuses on a disturbing situation or memory. Functional magnetic resonance imaging studies have shown that stimulating these acupuncture points affects the release of brain chemicals in ways that reduce pain and shut off the fight-or-flight response activated by emotional stress.[79]

The EFT technique is easily learned and can be readily practiced at home. If a problem is very complex or the person has been severely traumatized, it is advisable, at least initially, to work with a mental health professional when applying the treatment; this will yield better results.

Research Results

A randomized controlled study of veterans with PTSD found that six sessions of EFT coaching, in addition to primary care, reduced pain by an average of 41%. Anxiety and depression were also significantly reduced. The benefits of EFT treatment were maintained at the six-month follow-up.[80]

EFT treatment for chronic tension-type headache sufferers was evaluated in a randomized controlled study. Participants were taught the EFT method and instructed to use it twice daily for two months. The frequency and intensity of the headaches were significantly reduced in the intervention group. Quality of life and sleep also significantly improved.[81]

Another randomized controlled study examined the use of EFT for women with fibromyalgia who were out of work for at least three months. The treatment group participated in an eight-week EFT program administered over the Internet. Compared to a waitlist control group, the treated women had significantly less pain, anxiety, depression, and pain catastrophizing. The treated women also had significantly better vitality, social function, activity levels, and mental health, and fewer stress symptoms.[82]

A study of 194 health care professionals from varied occupations—including physicians, nurses, psychotherapists, chiropractors, psychiatrists, alternative medicine practitioners, and allied professionals—evaluated whether EFT had an effect on anxiety, depression, and other psychological symptoms. Participants engaged in a 90-minute EFT demonstration and self-application. On follow-up, three months later, overall symptom severity had dropped by 34%. Pain scores dropped by 68%; traumatic memories intensity dropped by 83%; and cravings dropped by 83%. More frequent subsequent EFT use was associated with a larger decrease in severity of symptoms at follow-up.[83]

In his book *The Tapping Solution for Pain Relief*, Nick Ortner, a leader in the EFT field, reported that he has seen thousands of people heal from chronic pain of all kinds using EFT. In his book, he described individuals who've healed from phantom limb pain,[84] fibromyalgia, chronic tooth pain/infection, and many other types of pain. His book gives specific instructions for applying the technique at home by focusing on the pain itself as well as possible underlying issues and emotions.[85]

A more general guide to EFT with instructions for personal use is available free at www.emofree.com.

Hypnosis

In the altered state of consciousness called hypnosis, the individual has increased receptivity to suggestion and the ability to modify perception and memory and to control physiological functions usually considered involuntary. These characteristic of the hypnotic altered state can be very useful in reducing pain.[86]

Psychologist Joseph Barber reported that it is a common misunderstanding that hypnosis achieves its effects in pain management by facilitating relaxation. Although relaxation suggestions are often part of the process for putting someone into a hypnotic state (called the induction), hypnosis is much more than a relaxed state. A hypnotic state can exist even when some indicators of arousal, such as blood pressure, are high.[87]

Hypnosis treatment begins with a hypnotic induction, a series of suggestions that alter the state of consciousness to a state accepting of suggestions. Induction involves eliciting the patient's attention and cooperation, suggesting a progressively narrower range of attention and directing attention inward, along with suggesting dissociation (a perceived detachment from emotions or the body). Once the hypnotic state has been achieved, suggestions are given for therapeutic change, such as increasing feelings of comfort during the session and afterward. Suggestions are then given for ending the experience, which usually incorporate suggestions for feeling well and alert.[88]

Hypnosis interventions strive to alter two aspects of the experience of pain, the sensory and the affective. The sensory component relates to the location and quality of the pain, including whether the pain is sharp or dull, burning or cold, aching or tingling, intermittent or constant. The affective component is about how much the pain bothers us and is related to what the pain means to us. This may include, for instance, whether we believe the pain indicates a life-threatening condition or is punishment for some wrongdoing.[89]

There has been considerable discussion within the field about receptivity to hypnotic suggestion. Some people are more "hypnotizable" than others are. Research in the field indicates that those who are more responsive to hypnotic suggestion are more likely to achieve a higher degree of pain reduction than those with low responsiveness. But even those with low responsiveness can achieve significant pain relief. Patients more responsive to suggestion seem to achieve relief in both the sensory and affective components of pain, whereas those with low suggestibility tend to achieve relief primarily in the affective component of pain.[90]

The first use of hypnosis was reported by Anton Mesmer in the 1700s. Mesmer announced that he was able to improve physical symptoms by inducing an altered state. A highly controversial figure, he was labeled a fraud by the authorities. Fifty years later, in the 1840s, a few British and Scottish surgeons began using hypnosis as a method of anesthesia during operations with great success, attracting widespread attention throughout Europe and the United States. Just a short time after that, chemical agents effective for anesthesia became available. They were easier and quicker to use than hypnosis; consequently, hypnotic techniques fell out of favor.[91]

Research Results

Over the years, interest has revived in hypnosis as a medicinal tool. It was endorsed in the 1950s by the British, Canadian, and American medical associations.[92] A review of controlled studies of the use of hypnosis for pain management, completed by researchers at the Mount Sinai Medical School in 2000, found a significant beneficial effect of hypnosis in the treatment of pain. The average patient receiving hypnosis treatment achieved greater pain relief than 75% of control subjects.[93] Another review of studies of hypnosis in the treatment of chronic pain for a broad range of medical conditions—including migraine headache, sickle cell disease, osteoarthritis, and fibromyalgia—was published in 2006. Hypnotic interventions were found to be more effective, on average, than no treatment and more effective than medical management or physical therapy. Other treatments that incorporated hypnotic-like suggestions, such as relaxation and biofeedback, were found to produce similar effects. Where studies looked at long-term effects, pain relief was found to last for up to 12 months.[94] There are no documented reports of long-term harm from hypnosis.[95]

Barriers to the Use of Mind/Body Treatments in Chronic Pain

Two main factors stand in the way of widespread use of mind/body techniques in chronic pain treatment: lack of awareness of their efficacy and a severe shortage of health care professionals trained in their use.

Mind/body techniques, more than any other approach, involve teaching the patient self-management. Once skills are learned, the patient may no longer need medical—including pharmacological—intervention. There are no big profits to be made and no large marketing budgets available to promote their use. Marketing campaigns for pharmaceutical and surgical interventions divert attention from these simple, safe, and effective tools.

While mental health professionals are best positioned to offer mind/body treatment approaches to chronic pain, they are, unfortunately, in severely short supply throughout most of the country. The federal government defines a mental health shortage area as one having fewer than one mental health provider of any kind for each 10,000 residents. Considering that 17% of the US population has a diagnosable mental illness in any one year, and 6% are severely mentally ill, this is a ludicrously low definition of shortage. Add to that the one in three Americans suffering from chronic pain, who might benefit from psychological intervention. Even with this inadequate definition of shortage, 93 million Americans currently live in geographic areas designated as a mental health shortage area.[96] In addition, few of the existing mental health professionals in the United States are trained in the use of mind/body techniques to treat chronic pain.

A major reason for the shortage of mental health providers is inadequate insurance reimbursement. Fees paid to nonphysician mental health providers who participate in health insurance networks have, for the most part, not increased in more than 35 years. Factoring in inflation, this means that the fees for mental health providers have decreased by about 66% from their value in the mid-1980s, while the cost of business expenses has risen. Few new college graduates can afford to become mental health clinicians, and existing providers are aging out of the field. In addition, those mental health providers who remain in practice are severely financially constrained from obtaining training in new techniques.

Chapter 6

Manipulative and Body-Based Practices

Chiropractic Treatment

The chiropractic profession was founded in the United States in 1895. Chiropractors diagnose, treat, and prevent disorders of the musculoskeletal system. More than 90% of patients who seek care from chiropractors are seeking relief from pain, including back and neck pain and headaches.[1]

In the United States, it takes a minimum of six years of university-level education to become a chiropractor. This includes two years of university credits in qualifying subjects and four years of undergraduate study at a chiropractic college. After completing their studies, would-be chiropractors must pass a state licensing exam. Chiropractors are licensed health care providers in all 50 states. They provide drug-free treatment, with an emphasis on manual treatments, including spinal manipulation.

Chiropractic treatment has been shown to be much safer than any conventional pain treatments. The estimated risk for serious complications for cervical (neck) manipulation is 6.39 per 10 million manipulations; for lumbar (low-back) manipulation, the estimate is 1 serious complication for every 100 million manipulations, according to a 1998 study sponsored by nonpartisan nonprofit research institute the

RAND Corporation. Compare this to the 156,000 serious complications per 10 million cervical spine surgeries and 32,000 serious complications per 10 million patients using nonsteroidal anti-inflammatory drugs (NSAIDs). The same literature review found that spinal manipulation was more effective for both acute and subacute low-back pain without sciatica than comparison treatments, and that cervical manipulation was effective for neck pain and muscle tension-type headaches.[2]

In 1997, the Agency for Health Care Policy and Research reported that chiropractic spinal manipulation was one of the few evidence-based treatments recommended for the treatment of low-back pain.[3] The World Health Organization (WHO) admitted the World Federation of Chiropractic, which represents national chiropractic associations from more than 70 countries, into official relations as a nongovernmental organization in 1997. This indicates that WHO considers chiropractic an accepted healing modality.

Between 1979 and 1999, treatment guidelines from governments around the world recognized chiropractic spinal manipulation as an effective treatment for low-back pain, including in the United States (1994);[4] Great Britain (1994);[5]Sweden (1987);[6] Denmark (1999);[7]Australia (1986);[8] and New Zealand (1979).[9]

Most studies have shown that chiropractic treatment saves money compared to conventional treatment for these conditions.[10] Despite all this, chiropractic treatment is still considered alternative medicine, and its use is actively discouraged by the US health care system.

AMA Attack

Since the founding of the chiropractic profession, the American Medical Association has actively worked to contain and eliminate the profession. During the first half of the 20th century, with the active encouragement of the AMA, many chiropractors were prosecuted for practicing medicine without a license—and many went to jail.

Dr. John Edwards has been a practicing chiropractor in upstate New York since 1959, four years before New York State finally licensed chiropractors. According to Edwards, judges would often preside over the conviction and sentencing of a chiropractor and then ask the chiropractor to meet them privately in their chambers, where they would request a spinal adjustment. When chiropractors went to jail, they were met with similar requests from the correction officers.[11] Eventually, all US states licensed chiropractors, beginning with Minnesota in 1905. The last was Louisiana in 1974.

Doyle Taylor was director of the AMA Department of Investigation, where he founded the Committee on Quackery in 1963. The committee had the avowed goal of creating a health care monopoly that would eliminate the chiropractic profession.[12] Because chiropractic made little use of technology and no use of drugs, the profession had no strong financial allies. Meanwhile, the AMA had access to the deep pockets of the pharmaceutical industry to further its goals.[13] AMA members faced expulsion from the association not only for referring to chiropractors but even for belonging to the same country club or church or synagogue—association was strictly prohibited.[14] As a result, chiropractors faced discrimination in not only their professional life but also their personal life.

In October 1976, Chester Wilk, DC, and four other chiropractors sued the American Medical Association for libel. The suit claimed that the defendants had participated for years in an illegal conspiracy to destroy chiropractic. The Wilk suit also included other powerful medical groups as codefendants, including the American Hospital Association, the American College of Surgeons, the American College of

Physicians, and the Joint Commission on Accreditation of Hospitals.

In 1987, after years of court battles, US District Court judge Susan Getzendanner found the AMA and its officials guilty of attempting to eliminate the chiropractic profession. It took 11 years of legal action, an effort most providers of alternative treatments would be unable to sustain, for a federal appellate court judge to rule that the AMA had engaged in a "lengthy, systematic, successful, and unlawful boycott" designed to restrict cooperation between MDs and chiropractors to eliminate the chiropractic profession as a competitor in the US health care system.

During the proceedings, evidence showed that the AMA attempted to

- undermine chiropractic schools;.
- undercut insurance programs for chiropractic patients.;
- conceal evidence of the effectiveness of chiropractic care.;
- subvert government inquiries into the effectiveness of chiropractic.; and
- promote other activities that would control the monopoly that the AMA had on health care.

The AMA claimed that physician treatment was superior to chiropractic; however, data presented from the Workmen's Compensation Bureau studies comparing chiropractic care to care by physicians showed that chiropractors were "twice as effective as medical physicians, for comparable injuries, in returning injured workers to work at every level of injury severity."

As part of the lawsuit settlement, the AMA was required to cease its efforts to restrict the professional association of chiropractors and AMA members. The AMA was also ordered to notify its 275,000 members of the court's decision. In addition, the American Hospital Association (AHA) was required to send out 440,000 notices informing hospitals that the AHA had no objection to the provision of chiropractic care in hospitals. The judgment was upheld by the 7th US Circuit Court of Appeals.[15]

Reduction in Access to Chiropractic Care

In the end, despite winning many victories in both the courts and the court of public opinion, chiropractors have had their practices severely restricted by organized medicine because of the advent of managed care. Patient access to chiropractic treatment is restricted by requirements for preapproval of care and limitations in length of care. The paperwork burden on chiropractors consumes a substantial, and unpaid, portion of their professional days. In addition, over the last 30 years, chiropractic fees have for the most part stayed the same or even decreased. Increases have been rare as well as minimal (10% or less). Consequently, the number of chiropractic jobs in the United States declined from 65,000 in the year 2000[16] to 44,400 in 2012.[17]

A study published in 2010 found that 10% of California chiropractors who were licensed in 1970 left the profession within 10 years of graduating from chiropractic school. That number rose to a peak of 27.8% for those who were licensed in 1991. The 10-year attrition rate remained between 20% and 25% for chiropractors licensed between 1992 and 1998. The authors of the study found that spiralling tuition costs and decreasing insurance reimbursement rates likely caused the increased attrition rates. Many chiropractors reported a 50% decrease in income owing to managed care.[18]

The percentage of the population utilizing chiropractic in a 12-month period more than doubled during the 1980s, to almost 10% of the US population,[19] then increased modestly during the 1990s to 11%.[20] The increase in patients was more than offset, however, by decreases in the number of visits per episode of care because of managed care restrictions.[21] By 2002, the chiropractic utilization rate had dropped to 7.5% .[22]

The opposite occurred in Germany, where reported chiropractor utilization rates increased significantly from 8.1% in a 1999 study[23] to 14.3% in a 2004 study.[24]

The Case of Dr. Lee Masterson

Lee Masterson, DC, has been a practicing chiropractor in Delmar, New York, for more than 30 years. He reports that he sees many patients with intransigent medical problems. Like many chiropractors, he is often the last stop for a patient before back surgery, or a patient's last hope after back surgery or other medical interventions have failed. He says, "I've treated many patients over the years who have been able to avoid back surgery and saved insurance companies tens of thousands of dollars per patient. Then when it comes to paying me four hundred dollars for a course of treatment, they balk."

Masterson reported that often the insurance company requires patients to pay the specialist co-pay for their chiropractic visits—and the specialist co-pay is higher than the allowed fee. As a result, the patient must pay the entire cost of chiropractic treatment out of pocket. Since chiropractic visits are often needed multiple times per week for an extended period, chiropractic visits have become unaffordable for many people. In New York State and many other states, insurance companies are mandated to pay for chiropractic care. However, so far this skirting of the law has gone unchallenged. Most chiropractors, according to Masterson, are too busy "working in the trenches" to take time out to fight the system. Masterson also reported that most managed care companies require a physician referral. Insurance companies count the physician visit as the treatment evaluation and often won't pay chiropractors for the comprehensive evaluation they must do before performing adjustments.

Masterson reports routinely putting in 50 to 60 hours a week to make an adequate living and complete paperwork requirements. When his children were growing up, he rarely saw them because he was working 12-hour days, ending his workday at 7:30 p.m. He would eat dinner with his family at 8 p.m. Still, he remains dedicated to his work and his patients. "My patients appreciate me," he said, "They are very grateful." Unfortunately, the insurance companies are not.

The Case of Dr. Sheryl Drake

A practicing chiropractor in Albany, New York, since 1997, Sheryl Drake, DC, works with her husband, also a chiropractor, in an interdisciplinary practice called Albany Multi Medicine. The practice also includes a physician and a physical therapist. Drake reports that the practice works with many chronic pain patients and focuses strongly on rehabilitation, in the sense not only of decreasing pain but also restoring function. Like Masterson, Drake reported that stagnation in fees; increased costs for the patient, which make care unaffordable for many; and an increasing paperwork burden make remaining in practice very difficult. She is the mother of small children but must work until 11 p.m. or later most nights doing paperwork. Changes in New York State workers' compensation law has doubled the amount of required paperwork in recent years. Recently, her practice manager told her that they really needed to stop seeing workers' compensation patients. Drake says, "How can we do that? Many of these patients, who do heavy manual labour, the blue-collar workers, are the salt of the earth. They keep everything running. And workers' compensation wants to throw them under the bus."

Drake also reported that Medicare has lowered fees while increasing the paperwork burden on chiropractors. After the service has been provided and billed, Medicare asks for treatment records before it issues payment. Although Medicare technically has no limit on chiropractic visits, in practice it rarely considers more than 8 to 12 visits medically necessary and denies coverage for any additional visits. Once the patient has improved a little, Medicare and other insurance providers consider any additional treatment "maintenance therapy" and refuse to cover it. This differs from medication treatment, which insurance companies are willing to pay for indefinitely in the absence of any additional improvement. Chiropractic patients often must deteriorate into another acute episode before they can get any additional care covered.

Drake reports that many of the chiropractors in her graduating class have stopped practicing, most likely because they couldn't make it financially. When asked why she and her husband continue despite all the difficulties, Drake simply replied, "We do it for the patient."

Diane

Diane DeGiovine, one of my social work colleagues in upstate New York, is very grateful to her chiropractor for giving her back her life. Diane needed a combination of conventional and alternative therapies to get well but initially had great difficulty getting the care she needed. Ten years ago she began having severe back pain. A neurologist she consulted ordered an MRI and found nothing. She then consulted several alternative providers, including a chiropractor and acupuncturist, with no relief. She received a pain injection from a physician who hit her sciatic nerve, sending her pain level "through the roof." After a while, Diane lost the use of her right leg. She made frantic calls to her neurologist, who refused to respond to her calls for five or six weeks because "he'd already found nothing."

Diane (cont.)

When these problems landed her in the emergency room, Diane was sent home with crutches and pain meds. During the time her neurologist was ignoring her pleas for help, she lost 15 pounds because of her pain. Finally, her neurologist agreed to see her for an appointment and scheduled exploratory surgery. As she was being wheeled into surgery, Diane told her neurologist that besides whatever was going on with her right leg, she felt that something was also wrong on the left and asked him to look at that while he was doing the surgery. He refused. The neurologist found a synovial cyst on her sciatic nerve on the right and removed it. Her sciatic pain returned shortly after the surgery. Her neurologist told her that if she persisted in her complaints, he would do a complete spinal fusion. Diane insisted on another MRI and took the results to Dr. Paul Cooper at NYU Medical Center. Diane said, "Doctor Cooper had a cracker jack radiologist look at the X-rays." The radiologist found she had a broken vertebrae and facet joint that was sliding around as she moved. In July 2006, she had a medically necessary spinal fusion. The problem could have caused spinal cord damage and paralysis if it had remained untreated. Cooper told her that he had no idea how the first surgeon had missed the problem once he went in to do the other surgery. In hindsight, Diane is glad that her first surgeon didn't do her fusion because she is "quite sure he would have screwed it up." Dr. Anthony Frompong performed the fusion and did an excellent job.

Diane (cont.)

About five or six weeks after the surgery, Diane started physical therapy, but after six weeks, Diane reported, "Something was just not right. I felt like I had a board across my back." A friend referred her to chiropractor Craig Nelson who aligned her spine and prescribed exercises and ultrasound treatment. At first, the treatment occurred three times a week. Now Diane goes every week or two to keep herself well. She also regularly goes to the gym to keep fit.

Eight years after her surgery, Diane says, "I am the most fit I have ever been, at age fifty-six."

Diane has had to pay for most of her chiropractic treatment out of pocket over the years, as her insurance company, stating she failed to progress, stopped paying.

In the first year of her treatment, her chiropractor was denied admission to the provider panel of her insurance company. The only payment Nelson received during that time was her co-pay. He never asked her to pay the difference.

Physical Therapy

Physical therapists treat people with medical problems that impair their ability to move and to function in their daily lives. After examining the patient, physical therapists develop an individualized treatment plan to increase mobility, reduce pain, improve function, and prevent disability.[25] Physical therapists use a variety of techniques, which include heat, cold, water, ultrasound, electrical stimulation, manual therapy, and exercise.[26]

Manual therapy is treatment performed primarily with the hands. Manual therapy can include massage; mobilization (movement to loosen tight tissue around a joint to improve flexibility and alignment); and manipulation (pressure applied to a joint with hands or a special device).[27] Exercise can include stretching, core-strengthening exercises, lifting weights, and walking. It may also include instruction in a home-exercise program.[28]

Physical therapists must have a master's or doctoral degree from an accredited physical therapy program and pass the National Physical Therapy exam. Physical therapists may also be board certified in specialty areas, such as orthopedic, geriatric, neurological, or pediatric physical therapy, which requires an additional one to three years of study.[29]

The use of physical therapy techniques dates back to the days of Hippocrates, who used massage and other manual therapies as well as water therapy to treat people in 460 BCE. In modern times, physical therapy came into widespread use during the polio epidemic of 1916 and then was used to treat soldiers injured during World War I.[30]

A physical therapy session usually includes one or more treatment modalities combined with education, advice, and exercise. Effective treatment includes informing the patient about his condition, challenging distorted beliefs about pain and disability, and encouraging self-management. This treatment complexity has posed a challenge to physical therapy research because looking at just one of the treatment modalities does not accurately represent what happens in a visit.[31]

The three stages of rehabilitation are as follows:

1. *Acute:* The treatment focus in the acute stage is reducing tissue injury through relative rest (not bed rest, which has been shown to make problems worse); the use of modalities such as heat, cold, electrical stimulation, and ultrasound; and starting exercise to promote range of motion.

2. *Recovery:* Once adequate tissue healing has occurred, the recovery stage treatment is initiated, which includes exercises to promote flexibility, strength, and normalized awareness of the body's movement and position in space. This

stage may also include massage, traction, stretching, and joint mobilization to continue to promote soft tissue flexibility and healing.

3. *Functional:* In this stage, the focus is on regaining normal movement patterns and postures that may have been altered by the patient's efforts to compensate for chronic mechanical problems or injury.[32]

Research Results

A review of randomized controlled trials from 1961 to 2009 found strong evidence for the use of manual therapies in the treatment of chronic low-back pain and knee pain for adults with musculoskeletal pain. The authors also found studies reporting improvement in patients with fibromyalgia and neck and shoulder pain, but concluded that the quantity and quality of evidence was insufficient to draw conclusions about effectiveness of physical therapy for these conditions.[33]

Worsening Access to Physical Therapy

Health insurers usually limit coverage for physical therapy to a specific number of sessions per year (typically 20) or a limited period (typically 60 days). Medicare has a dollar limit of $1,900 per year for physical therapy. Insurers usually require preauthorization of physical therapy to determine if it is "medically necessary." This translates to extensive paperwork burdens for providers, with patients often having access to even fewer treatment sessions than their insurance contracts imply.

One large, multisite clinic in Spokane, Washington, reported that the average length of care for their patients was only 6.8 visits as a result of insurance restrictions, a situation that has worsened over the past decade.[34] This has occured despite studies showing that longer length of treatment is associated with better outcomes.[35]

Another worsening trend is that patients are required to pay higher co-pays, often a specialist co-pay of $30 to $40 per visit, which can exceed the allowed fee for the service. Like many other nonphysician providers, physical therapists have not received increases in fees in over 30 years.[36] High out-of-pocket cost for patients often prevent access to care.

Access to physical therapy care is expected to worsen because of provider shortages. The US Bureau of Labor Statistics has projected a 36% growth (73,500 positions) in the need for physical therapists from 2012 to 2022, mostly because of an aging population. This compares to an average projected growth for all occupations of 11% during the same time.[37] The American Physical Therapy Association projects a shortage of 41,000 physical therapists by 2020.

The Case of Dick Marrone

Dick Marrone, who retired in 2005, began working as a physical therapist in a hospital setting in 1972. He then worked in nursing homes, later establishing a part-time private practice. Marrone reported that when he first started working as a physical therapist, there were no set limits on care. Physicians prescribed physical therapy and reevaluated the medical necessity regularly. Insurance companies did not demand treatment notes or set limits on the length of care. Over time, treatment restrictions and paperwork burdens grew. In some situations, care was so limited by HMOs that Marrone would provide up to eight sessions of care free to ensure that a patient received an adequate course of treatment. Marrone retired earlier than he might otherwise have because of the difficulties of dealing with insurance companies.[38]

The Case of Michelle Kelleher

Michelle Kelleher, who maintains a private practice in Delmar, New York, started working as a physical therapist in 1966, initially working with children in hospital settings in New York City, Vermont, Seattle, and Albany. In 1985, she established her private practice. Kelleher reported that when HMOs came on the scene in the 1990s, fees were cut by 33% and have not been raised since. Typically, only six visits would be approved initially, and she would have to argue for more. Kelleher dropped the HMOs after five or six years and today has many self-pay clients. The innovative techniques she uses are often not reimbursed by insurance. Kelleher reported she knows of many physical therapists who have stopped practicing because of inadequate pay.[39]

The Case of John Grazione

John Grazione is past president of the pain management special interest group of the American Physical Therapy Association. He practices in Norwich, in western New York. He is 65 years old, has been in practice for 41 years, and works 11-to-12-hour days. Having to repeatedly justify care to insurance companies takes significant time from seeing patients and sometimes becomes so onerous that Grazione sees patients for the price of the co-pay alone. Grazione loves what he does and is much in demand. Many patients travel 50 to 60 miles several times a week to see him, and he has a four- to six-week waiting list for new patients. Providing the intensive hands-on care he believes his patients need while still making a living necessitates that he work long hours. Grazione plans to keep up his current pace for another five years and then reduce his work schedule to eight-hour days, which he says will be "like Club Med" for him.

Grazione says that because most insurances pay a set fee for a physical therapy visit, regardless of the time spent or the number of modalities used, many physical therapists cope with stagnant fees by spending less time with patients and doing less hands-on care so they can cram in more patients. He knows of other physical therapy practices that have simply folded or the therapists have gone to work for hospitals for a salary. Hospitals get paid higher fees because they are in a better position than individual practitioners to negotiate with insurance companies. Other physical therapists Grazione knows have gone to cash-only practices, so that their services are available only to those with higher incomes.[40]

Grazione reports that the debt burden on a new physical therapist makes financial survival even more difficult now than it was for older generations. Physical therapists are now required to have doctorates, with no pay increase to compensate. Grazione had to earn his doctorate after 30 years in practice. He reported that he has a new 23-year-old associate in his practice who will be paying on her student debt until she is 50 years old. People become physical therapists because they're passionate about what they do, not because they're going to become rich doing it, Grazione says.[41]

Therapeutic Massage and Other Forms of Bodywork

Therapeutic massage and bodywork include a wide variety of techniques that involve manipulation of soft tissue or subtle energy to alleviate pain or resolve structural imbalances so that health and well-being are improved.[42]

Physical therapists, chiropractors, and other types of health care providers may incorporate massage as one of the treatment modalities used during a session. Massage is also used as a stand-alone treatment, in which case the massage is usually of longer duration and more intensive.

As of 2014, there were 300,000 to 350,000 massage therapists and massage school students in the United States.[43] Forty-four states and the District of Columbia regulate massage therapists or provide voluntary state certification. In states that regulate massage therapy, massage therapists need have a minimum number of hours of training and pass an exam to practice.[44]

A survey found that 15% of adult Americans received at least one massage between July 2013 and July 2014. Of those visiting massage therapists, 54% had massage for medical reasons—such as pain management, rehabilitation of an injury, or overall wellness—and 92% agreed that massage can be effective in reducing pain.[45]

There are many different types of massage and bodywork. These can be classified into four types of approaches:

1. *Gentle bodywork* includes light application of touch, as in Swedish massage, craniosacral therapy, and lomi lomi massage. These techniques help the body relax and return to its natural state of balance. For treatment of pain, gentle bodywork techniques are best suited to patients in significant pain, at least initially, as they are less likely to aggravate the condition than forms of massage that use more pressure.

2. *Structural bodywork* includes Rolfing, Hellerwork, and other schools of structural integration. The goal of this bodywork is to change structure by creating a direct change in muscles, tendons, ligaments, and other soft tissues to restore structural balance and reduce strain. The pressure applied with these techniques can create short-term pain.

3. *Deep tissue bodywork,* which focuses on the alleviation of pain and discomfort, includes, in addition to deep tissue massage, neuromuscular

therapy, Trager psychophysical integration, and myofascial release.

4. *Movement therapy, or reeducation,* includes the Feldenkrais method, the Alexander technique, and Rolf movement work. Movement therapy aims to alter the person's habitual body usage to reduce muscle strain. Movement therapy also helps maintain the results of structural bodywork.[46]

Research Results

The research on therapeutic massage and bodywork is highly variable. Some of the published studies have small sample sizes, lack control groups, or fail to adequately describe the type or duration of the bodywork intervention. In some studies, it appears that the massage or bodywork intervention was provided by someone without adequate training. Nonetheless, numerous studies have shown that massage is a safe and effective treatment for chronic pain.

A 2001 study of patients with chronic low-back pain found that 10 massage sessions significantly reduced pain and disability, with benefits still evident 9 to 10 months after completions of treatment.[47]

A 2006 randomized study comparing up to 10 therapeutic massages over 10 weeks to use of a self-care book for chronic neck pain found that those in the massage group were significantly more likely to report improvement in function, how bothered they were by symptoms, and medication usage at the end of treatment. Sixteen weeks later, the massage treatment group still had better function, but the difference in symptoms bothering them had evaporated.[48]

A 2006 randomized controlled study of adults with osteoarthritis compared eight weeks of therapeutic massage (two massages per week for four weeks and then one massage weekly for four weeks) to usual care. There were significant reductions in pain, stiffness, and function in the massage group at the end of treatment, which generally persisted eight weeks after completion of treatment.[49]

A 2008 Cochrane Collaboration review of 13 randomized trials of massage for low-back pain, which included a total of 1,596 participants, concluded that massage was more likely to work when combined with exercises (usually stretching) and education, and that the benefits outweighed those achieved by relaxation, physical therapy, education in self-care, or acupuncture. Acupressure, or pressure point massage techniques, seemed to provide greater relief than Swedish massage did.[50]

A large 2011 randomized controlled study compared two types of massage—structural and relaxation—to usual care for people 20 to 65 years old with nonspecific chronic low-back pain. The treatment groups received 10 massages over a 10-week period by experienced massage therapists. Both massage groups had similar functional outcomes and symptom bothersomeness scores that were significantly superior to usual care. Benefits persisted for at least six months.[51]

A 2014 study comparing the effects of deep tissue massage on low-back pain to deep tissue massage plus NSAIDs found that 10 deep tissue massages of 30 minutes each effectively reduced low-back pain and associated disability. No additional benefit was seen from adding NSAIDs to the treatment.[52]

A 2014 systematic review of 10 randomized and nonrandomized controlled trials investigating the effectiveness of massage for fibromyalgia found that myofascial release resulted in large reductions in pain and moderate reductions in anxiety and depression. Improvements in fatigue, stiffness, and quality of life were also noted. Shiatsu massage was found to have similar positive benefits, while Swedish massage did not appear to benefit fibromyalgia patients.[53]

Another 2014 systematic review of nine randomized controlled studies of massage for fibromyalgia reached similar conclusions: massage therapy with a duration of at least five weeks improved pain, anxiety, and depression in fibromyalgia patients.[54]

Massage is a safe and effective treatment for many types of chronic pain. Unfortunately, most health insurance won't cover it. If the pain is caused by a work-related injury or auto accident, workers' compensation or auto insurance may cover massage.

Rolfing

My favorite type of bodywork is structural integration, which was developed by Ida Rolf, a biochemist, in the mid-20th century. Structural integration (SI) is also known as Rolfing.

More of My Story

Several years after resolving my disabling back pain problem, I developed a sharp pain in my left foot when I walked. It was diagnosed as a bone spur in my big toe joint. After more conservative treatments failed to address the problem, I had foot surgery to remove the bone spur. Shortly after the surgery, I developed a different kind of pain when I tried to walk. I could not walk more than a couple of blocks without being in agony. I could not stand for more than a few minutes or even set my foot on the floor when I was sitting without feeling severe pain. I consulted many medical practitioners, none of whom seemed to know what was wrong. The mind/body and other approaches I had used to successfully address my back pain were useless in resolving my foot pain.

More of My Story (cont.)

The pain persisted for 14 years, until someone suggested I try Rolfing. After two sessions, I felt as if I had a new foot.

Over the 20 years since, whenever I have developed pain that did not remit within a short time with the self-care strategies I have learned, I have booked a Rolfing session. For the last 13 years, these sessions have been with Allan Davidson. Allan was one of Ida Rolf's first trainees. Rolfing always helps.

Rolfing involves bringing the body as a whole into balance, rather than treating specific symptoms. For Rolfers, the essential question may be not what's wrong but where is it coming from and what's feeding it. Rolfing reduces biomechanical strain by promoting an optimal relationship of the body in gravity, through releasing and balancing the muscles and fascia of the body, and helping the body find more support.[55] Rolf also believed that SI would improve psychological well-being.[56]

During a Rolfing session, the practitioner applies manual force to the soft tissue in a more gradual and prolonged way than is typical of chiropractic manipulation, and with more pressure than is usual for massage. Sometimes the client is asked to perform slow movements as the pressure is applied to release stuckness in the myofascial tissues. Treatment also includes postural and movement awareness exercises. Transient pain can occur during the treatment. There can also be short-lived increases in anxiety or other negative emotions that spontaneously resolve within hours or days. The latter typically results in lasting improvements in levels of anxiety and depression.[57]

Rolf developed a series of 10 treatments that constitute the initial course of therapy. Each session focuses on specific biomechanical changes that contribute to the overall goal of freeing the body to find support in gravity. More advanced work is then possible.[58]

Research Results

Very few studies of structural integration have been conducted. Two retrospective case reviews have concluded that structural integration can reduce pain and improve function. A retrospective case review examined SI treatment of 20 cases of chronic musculoskeletal pain lasting an average of more than three years. After an average of eight sessions, 84.6% had improved range of motion, 73.7% had decreased pain, and 74.5% had improved function. Some 79% of patients rated themselves as improved.[59] A retrospective review of treatment of 31 people with chronic neck pain and stiffness who received 10 SI sessions found statistically significant improvements in range of motion and reductions in pain.[60]

David

David Delaney is a Rolfer whose own experience led him to become a practitioner. At the age of 17, David broke his leg very badly. He was in a hip cast for a long time. When his cast was removed, his leg "looked like a mackerel." David first tried massage and then Rolfing to get well. The Rolfing made a significant difference in his pain and functioning. An aspiring singer, David found that the Rolfing also helped his voice. When David started his Rolfing practice, he mainly worked with singers in the New York City area. Later he expanded his practice to the general public and eventually moved his practice to Colorado.

David's Rolfing practice allowed him to see how people hold trauma in the connective tissue of their bodies. Rolfing lets them release that. David reports that people's unprocessed memories are "in the fiber of their being."

> ## David (cont.)
>
> David eventually added other therapies to his practice. He became a licensed mental health counselor, a cranial sacral therapist, and a neurofeedback practitioner—a one-man interdisciplinary clinic. Unfortunately for many, David recently retired.[61]

Neuromuscular Therapy

Neuromuscular therapy (NMT), developed in England in the 1930s by Dr. Stanley Lief, uses static pressure to manipulate muscles, tendons, and connective tissue to balance the central nervous system and relieve pain. NMT addresses these five causes of pain:

1. *Ischemia*, a lack of blood supply to the soft tissue that causes hypersensitivity to touch
2. *Trigger points,* which are irritated points in the muscles that refer pain to other parts of the body
3. *Nerve compression, or entrapment,* as a result of bone, cartilage, or soft tissue creating pressure on a nerve
4. Postural imbalance
5. *Biomechanical dysfunction*, which results when an imbalance of the musculoskeletal system causes dysfunctional movement patterns

Neuromuscular therapy also promotes release of endorphins.[62]

The neuromuscular therapist uses thumbs, fingers, and elbows to release tissues in layers, from superficial to deep. The origins of the muscle pain as well as muscle insertions and the belly of the muscle are treated. The therapist identifies the constrictions and trigger points by touch and then applies an appropriate amount of pressure to resolve the problem. Patients are encouraged to drink adequate amounts of water; supplement with multivitamins, B-12, and B-6; and do stretching exercises to further enhance the therapy.[63]

Chapter 7

Nutritional Interventions

Decades of research have shown that diet plays an important role in chronic pain. The human body constantly makes new cells to replace aging or damaged cells. These cells, the building blocks of our tissues and organs, require certain foods and nutrients for healthy development; other foods and substances are detrimental to cell development. In addition, the nutrients we ingest are the raw ingredients for our hormones, neurotransmitters, digestive enzymes, and other essential substances that keep our bodies healthy and in balance. Changing what you eat can have a significant impact on your pain levels.

A whole-foods diet that emphasizes fresh fruits and vegetables, whole grains, and lean meats reduces pain and inflammation. Processed foods and sugars and unhealthy fats increase pain and inflammation.[1] In addition, certain nutritional supplements—including omega-3 fatty acids, B vitamins, vitamin D, magnesium, and antioxidants—also have pain-reducing properties. There is considerable scientific evidence that certain foods are as effective at reducing pain as medications.[2]

One survey of 50 chronic pain patients receiving long-term opioid therapy at a suburban chronic pain clinic found that their diets were extremely unhealthy. They consumed an average of two servings of fruits and vegetables per day (compared to the recommended five or more servings). The average vitamin D intake was only 244 IU daily (compared to a recommended intake of 2000 to 8000 IU). Average added sugars were 74.5 grams a day[3] (compared to the maximum of 25 grams per day total of sugar recommended by the World Health Organization[4]).

Antioxidants

Antioxidants are substances that protect cells against damage from free radicals. Flavonoids are very powerful antioxidants that reduce inflammation and strengthen connective tissue in joints. Flavonoids, can be found in many fruits and vegetables and other plant-derived foods, including broccoli, blueberries, grapefruit, onions, apples, oranges, soybeans, chocolate, pomegranates, limes, lemons, tomatoes, carrots, red wine, and tea.[5]

Other antioxidants that reduce inflammation are vitamins C and E, selenium, and carotenoids. Foods high in vitamin C include citrus fruits, cabbage, strawberries, red bell peppers, and kiwis. Nuts, seeds, avocados, and olive oil are good food sources of vitamin E.[6] As with many nutrients, it can be difficult to get adequate, much less optimal, amounts of these nutrients in the diet. These antioxidants can also be found in nutritional supplements.

Essential Fatty Acids

Omega-3 and omega-6 fatty acids also have anti-inflammatory properties, though they must be ingested in proper proportion or omega-6 fatty acids can promote inflammation. The typical American diet contains 20 to 50 times more omega-6 fatty acids than omega-3 fatty acids—when the ideal ratio is 1:1.[7] The frequent consumption of processed foods containing omega-6 fatty acids in the form of hydrogenated vegetable oils, also known as trans fats, is a large part of the problem. Food sources of omega-3 fatty acids include fatty fish; flax seeds; walnuts; and olive, grapeseed, primrose, borage, and walnut oils.[8] Omega-3 fatty acids are also readily available in supplement form.

In a 2006 study, 125 neurology patients with neck or back pain took 1200 mg or 2400 mg per day of omega-3 essential fatty acids for an average of 75 days. Sixty percent rated their overall pain as improved; 60% rated their joint pain as improved; and 59% had discontinued their NSAID prescription medications. Some 80% said they were satisfied with their improvement, and 88% said they would continue to take the supplement.[9]

A randomized controlled study of 56 chronic headache patients found that increasing omega-3 EFAs and decreasing omega-6 EFAs for 12 weeks reduced headache pain and the number of headache days per month, along with improving overall quality of life.[10]

A meta-analysis of 10 randomized controlled trials of the use of omega-3s with rheumatoid arthritis patients found that dosages of greater than 2.7 g a day for longer than three months significantly reduced the use of NSAIDs. There was also a trend toward a reduction in tender points, swollen joints, and morning stiffness, along with improved physical function in the patients who supplemented with omega-3s.[11]

A study of patients with inflammatory bowel disease found that supplementation with omega-3 fatty acids favorably altered the composition of the cell membranes and was associated with disease remission.[12]

According to Dr. Joseph Maroon, a board-certified neurosurgeon who practices at the University of Pittsburgh Medical Center, omega-3s use the same pathways to block inflammation that NSAIDs do, but they do it more safely with far fewer side effects. Maroon became interested in using omega-3s after he developed an ulcer treating his own joint and muscle pain with NSAIDs. He later coauthored a book, *Fish Oil: The Natural Anti-inflammatory*.[13]

Vitamin D

Recent research has shown that vitamin D plays an extremely important role in chronic pain and that many people are at high risk for vitamin D deficiency. Levels of the vitamin can be measured with a simple blood test. Levels below 20 ng/mL (50 nmol/L) are generally considered deficient in conventional medicine. Others have defined deficiency as below 32 ng/mL, with the optimum range 50 to 70 ng/mL.[14]

Vitamin D is produced naturally in the body when the skin is exposed to ultraviolet rays from sunlight. Using sunscreen blocks the body's ability to produce vitamin D. People with dark skin synthesize 99% less vitamin D because melanin, the substance responsible for dark skin pigmentation, absorbs the UVB rays. Our bodies also become less able to synthesize vitamin D as we age. People living in the northern United States, where the sun is less direct and winters are longer, are also less likely to synthesize enough of the vitamin.[15] Many drugs also block the synthesis of vitamin D or reduce absorption, including some antacids, barbiturates, anticonvulsants, antirejection drugs, antiviral drugs, nicotine, blood thinners, cholesterol-lowering medication, and steroids.[16]

Food sources of this critical vitamin include fortified milk, egg yolk, cod liver oil, oysters, fatty fish, fortified soy milk, and fortified cereal.[17] These foods, however, are rarely consumed in sufficient quantities to maintain vitamin D at optimum levels. For instance, to obtain a target dose of 4000 to 8000 IU of vitamin D a day, a person would need to consume ¼ cup of cod-liver oil daily or 18 to 36 capsules.[18] Fortunately, vitamin D is inexpensive and readily available in supplement form. Vitamin D3, the natural form of vitamin D, is absorbed more readily than the synthetic form, vitamin D2.[19, 20]

Research Results

A study at the University of Minnesota of people with nonspecific musculoskeletal pain (pain without evidence of injury, disease, or anatomical or neurological defect) found that 93% of participants were deficient in vitamin D.[21] Another study, this one including participants with nonspecific musculoskeletal pain from diverse age groups and ethnicities, found that 100% of African American, Hispanics, and Native Americans were vitamin D deficient. All subjects younger than 30 were also deficient, with 55% severely so and five patients so deficient that their vitamin D levels were undetectable.[22]

Other studies in adults have shown that an inadequate level of vitamin D is associated with many other types of pain:[23]

- Nonspecific bone and joint pain
- Fatigue
- Muscle weakness
- Fibromyalgia
- Osteoarthritis
- Rheumatoid disorders
- Headaches
- Cardiovascular disorders
- Immune disorders
- Depression
- Chronic fatigue syndrome

A 2014 review of vitamin D status and ill health found that low vitamin D concentrations were associated with the following:[24]

- Cardiovascular disease
- High cholesterol levels
- Inflammation
- Diabetes
- Weight gain
- Infectious diseases
- Multiple sclerosis
- Mood disorders
- Declining cognitive function
- Physical functional impairment
- Colorectal cancer
- Mortality from all causes

Many studies have documented a reduction in pain when vitamin D supplements have been given to people in chronic pain. An article published in *Archives of Internal Medicine* reported that five patients who had chronic pain and low vitamin D levels had resolution of their pain in five to seven days after they were given vitamin D2 supplements. These patients had been hypersensitive to pain stimuli, and the pain did not improve with the use of any pain medications, including narcotics and tricyclic antidepressants. One of the patients had a decline in vitamin D level and a return of pain after several months; the pain was again resolved with vitamin D supplementation.[25]

A randomized controlled trial in the Netherlands of vitamin D3 supplementation of nonspecific musculoskeletal pain in non-Western (Arab and African) immigrants found that patients receiving a single dose of 150,000 IU of vitamin D3 were more likely, after six weeks, to report pain relief and an improvement in ability to climb stairs than those in the placebo group. Those receiving a second dose of vitamin D3 at six weeks were more likely to report improvements than the group that didn't receive a second dose.[26]

A randomized controlled study of patients with knee pain and vitamin D insufficiency, who received either vitamin D supplementation or a placebo for a year, found that the treatment group experienced significantly less pain and better knee function than the placebo group.[27] US veterans with multiple areas of chronic pain and low vitamin D levels who were given vitamin D supplementation had less pain, better sleep, and better quality of life.[28]

A randomized double-blind study of children and adolescents with sickle cell disease given a six week course of high-dose vitamin D found that the treatment group had fewer pain days per week and higher physical quality of life scores over a period of 6 months.[29]

A small study of women with diabetes who had neuropathic pain, tingling, and numbness found that six months of weekly vitamin D2 supplementation reduced pain and depression.[30]

A 2011 editorial in the *Scandinavian Journal of Primary Health Care* stated that vitamin D supplementation in patients with chronic pain seems reasonable, as the treatment is cheap and relatively safe, and evidence indicates that vitamin D supplementation has overall positive effects on health. The editorial recommended a daily dose of 2000 IU for chronic pain patients.[31] Others have documented a vitamin D requirement of 4000 to 8000 IU daily, or 35 IU per pound of body weight.[32] A more individualized approach, based on testing of vitamin D levels along with follow-up testing to determine the level of supplementation needed to maintain adequate blood serum levels, would probably yield the most effective results.

Despite the plethora of evidence accumulating on widespread vitamin D deficiency, the large number of chronic and life-threatening conditions preventable and treatable with vitamin D supplementation, and the safety and low cost of vitamin D testing and supplementation, in June 2014, the US Preventive Services Task Force declined to endorse screening for vitamin D deficiency in healthy adults. In its report, the task force cited insufficient evidence of benefit.[33]

Dr. Joseph Mercola, a well-known holistic physician, recommends also supplementing with vitamin K2 if you are taking vitamin D supplements. Vitamin K2 helps keep calcium where it belongs in the body. The only known toxicity from excessive vitamin D intake is related to excessive calcium in the bloodstream.[34]

Magnesium

Magnesium is another nutrient that has been shown to be helpful in treating many different types of chronic pain, including low-back pain, headache, complex regional pain syndrome, fibromyalgia, and sickle cell disease.

Research Results

A 2012 randomized controlled study of magnesium in the treatment of chronic low-back pain with a neuropathic component (with degenerative disc or nerve compression) found that two weeks of daily intravenous magnesium infusion (1 g of magnesium sulfate) followed by four weeks of oral magnesium capsules (magnesium oxide 400 mg plus magnesium gluconate 100 mg twice daily) significantly reduced pain intensity and improved lumbar spine range of motion. The improvements were present throughout the 6-week treatment period and were still present at 6 months.[35]

A 2013 study found that supplementation with 300 mg/day of magnesium citrate in fibromyalgia patients decreased the number of tender points and improved functioning, mood, pain, and fatigue after eight weeks. Higher magnesium serum levels were associated with less severe symptoms.[36]

A 2009 pilot study evaluated the use of intravenous magnesium in patients with complex regional pain syndrome. Five days of intravenous magnesium sulfate (3 g/100 lbs of body weight) significantly improved pain and quality of life and reduced impairment. Benefits were still present at 12 weeks.

A small 2005 study found that two months of oral magnesium supplements reduced chronic and episodic tension-type headache frequency in children by an average of over 80%, improvements persisting at six-month and one-year follow-ups. The study used an easily absorbable form of magnesium called magnesium pidolate at a dosage level of 2.25 g twice per day.

A study of sickle cell disease patients who were given 540 mg of magnesium pidolate daily for six months found the median number of painful days in a six-month period decreased from 15 in the year before the trial to one during the six-month trial period.[37]

Susanne

In 1996, Susanne Stratton developed severe pain in her left shoulder. X-rays showed nothing, and doctors never offered an MRI. For four years, she tried a variety of treatments— physical therapy, cortisone shots, anti-inflammatory drugs, ultrasound treatments. Nothing helped. She could not work or sleep because of the pain.

Susanne (cont.)

Finally, she was able to obtain an MRI, which showed a severe rotator cuff tear, a bone spur, and a deltoid muscle that was abnormally positioned. She had surgery to correct the abnormalities. But she woke up from the surgery in tremendous pain and with a paralyzed left arm. She was diagnosed with reflex sympathetic dystrophy (now called complex regional pain syndrome, or CRPS).

Susanne was told she would never use her left arm again. She continued with weekly physical therapy and occupational therapy. The pain was excruciating. Her daily life consisted of violent shaking on the left side of her body (including her neck and head) if she attempted to lift or move her left arm.

In 2000, she was referred to a pain management specialist who wanted to give her injections that would numb her from her neck down to her fingers. She was not comfortable with him or his recommendations, so she didn't follow through with his medical advice.

After being out of work for a full year because of her disability, she was financially strained and became sicker from all of the stress. Side effects from the narcotic pain medications negatively affected her ability to function on a daily basis. She was nauseous and depressed and experienced cloudy thinking.

The following year, Susanne was diagnosed with a prediabetic condition and had a precancerous pap smear. She was also experiencing reoccurring fevers reaching 103°F. At this point, a friend referred Susanne to Dr. Arta Salma, a naturopath. Salma told Susanne to throw everything away in her kitchen and purchase a Champion juicer.

Salma changed Susanne's nutritional intake to nothing but fruits and vegetables and suggested an all-alkalized diet. Nothing was to be eaten from a box or a can. No dairy or meat. No breads or processed foods.

Susanne (cont.)

She was told to live on raw fruits and vegetables and plant sources of protein, including avocados, almonds, and flaxseed and coconut oils, which support and create an alkalized body. Susanne learned that an alkalized body cannot produce disease. If the body's pH balance is too acidic, it compromises the immune system. Susanne's pH level was a −5, the worst level possible. The ideal pH is 7. Susanne's goal was to become alkalized and reach a pH level of 7.

Eventually, Susanne was released to go back to work part time using only her one good arm. She continued her fruit and vegetable intake, along with daily juicing using her Champion juicer. After four months with her nutritional changes, Susanne had reached a pH level of seven, had reversed her precancerous cells, and was no longer prediabetic. After six months, Susanne regained some movement in her shoulder. After 13 months, she had complete movement in her left arm, and the pain was gone. She is pain free to this day.

In 2010, Susanne had surgery on her right shoulder for a torn ligament. This time, she healed in half the time because her body was so healthy.

Susanne still follows a mostly raw diet today. She has gone back to school, studying at the Wellness Forum Institute in Ohio, and has become a nutritional educator, a certified health coach, and a wellness coordinator. Furthermore, she is a senior sales coordinator with NSA and Juice Plus+. Juice Plus+ is a "whole-food" supplement consisting of 17 different dehydrated fruits and vegetables in a capsule. It is also available in gummies.

For Susanne, changing her nutrition, juicing, and living on raw fruits and vegetable, along with Juice Plus+, has been pivotal in helping her get well. [38]

Censorship of Health Claims for Food and Supplements

You may be very surprised as you read about the significant benefits of food and nutritional supplements in the treatment of chronic pain. You may wonder why you haven't heard about these benefits before or why your doctor doesn't know about them. The reason is that it is a crime for food or supplement producers to make any claims about the health benefits of their products.

According to constitutional lawyer Jonathan Emord, making a claim that a product treats disease without securing government preapproval of the product as a drug is, universally, a crime. Offenders can face prison terms equivalent to a life sentence. The sale of the products can be prohibited, and the products can be seized and destroyed. Few, if any, food or supplement producers can afford the hundreds of millions of dollars it costs to get drug approval. When a producer makes health claims for nutritional products, it's a crime regardless of whether the information is true or is supported by scientific evidence.[39] In the United States, the law that contains these provisions is the Dietary Supplement Health and Education Act (DSHEA) of 1994.

According to Emord, this censorship results in an unequal playing field in which therapeutic claims can be made for pharmaceuticals but not for foods and nutritional supplements. This leads consumers to develop the distorted view that only pharmaceuticals can prevent or treat disease, and it gives the drug companies an unfair competitive advantage.[40]

Drug regulators who are political appointees are richly rewarded for their efforts favoring drug companies. They commonly overrule the safety concerns expressed by medical reviewers within the career bureaucracy, as was seen in the approval of Zohydro described earlier. When these political appointees leave office, they secure lucrative positions with the companies they formerly regulated.[41]

Emord sued the FDA on behalf of multiple plaintiffs for censorship of health claims. In 1999, the US Court of Appeals for the DC Circuit in *Pearson v. Shalala* ruled that the FDA's absolute censorship of health claims for nutritional products was a violation of the First Amendment. The court required the FDA to allow non-FDA-approved claims on product labels while relying on claims qualification ("These claims have not been evaluated by the FDA") instead of suppressing all claims.[42] This decision and several subsequent other cases filed because of violations of the initial decision have not resolved the situation, according to Emord, because the FDA refuses to adhere to the court's orders.[43]

Attempts to Discredit Nutritional Research and Restrict Access to Supplements

Scientists all over the world are producing more and more evidence that nutrients, particularly in large doses, can heal disease. As this evidence continues to accumulate, the need for pharmaceutical companies to defend against this information to protect their profits becomes ever more pressing.[44]

In recent years, a host of articles has shown results that conflict with long-standing proof of nutritional benefits in preventing and managing disease. For example, they have shown that low-fat diets don't prevent heart disease or that antioxidant vitamins don't prevent cancer. A close examination of these studies reveals that they were designed to fail. For instance, the study of low-fat diets showed too little reduction of fat intake in the "low-fat" group to be meaningful; likewise, the dosages of antioxidants in the cancer studies weren't large enough to have an impact. It's no surprise that these studies are typically funded by groups with a strong conflict of interest, and that they are widely circulated to the media.

The Alliance for Natural Health (ANH) is at the forefront in advocating for consumer access to supplements and in exposing the disinformation campaign against natural foods and supplements. ANH is an international nongovernmental organization based in the United Kingdom. It was founded in 2002 to protect and promote natural and sustainable approaches to health care. The ANH is of the opinion that today's dominant Western medical model relies too heavily on the use of pharmaceutical drugs, and that the use of natural health care is a fundamental human right that governments should not interfere with. The alliance is working to help facilitate the development of scientific and legal frameworks for natural health care. ANH–USA, in Washington, D.C., is its US affiliate.

Dr. Robert Verkerk is founder as well as scientific and executive director of ANH. Some of his agency's time and resources are devoted to investigating negative vitamin studies to determine if they were designed to fail. Verkerk reports,

> We see far too much of the wrong vitamin being used or too little of the right one being used or a combination of the two. We are also seeing a number of clinical studies that were conducted in the 1990's and early 2000's that are reappearing by the way of systematic reviews and meta-analyses. When we look at these studies of studies, we see peculiar selection decisions related to which studies to include and which ones to exclude. And they have been timed to keep these studies in people's minds at a time when an international regulating system

designed to limit our access to natural health care products is ramping up.

Verkerk also reports that many of the vitamins used in these studies are produced by pharmaceutical companies—not members of the natural products industry. "They deliver isolated vitamins that are synthetic forms that behave in a very different fashion than when they are delivered as natural complexes," Verkerk says.

Verkerk believes that there are many situations in which researchers intentionally try to produce negative results in vitamin studies.

> I think that you have another system where companies fund the trials, produce the vitamins for the trials, and then make damn sure that the results of the trials, when they are negative, get on the front page of the newspapers. I think there is certainly an agenda there. All you need is about six large clinical trials that deliver either no results or adverse findings in relation to vitamins. Then you need three or four meta-analyses that keep on confirming those results over and over again. That is what has been done, and it is the perfect vehicle required to justify massive tightening up of the regulatory regime around supplements. We're seeing this all over the world. In Canada, these kinds of studies have generated the National Health Products Regulation of 2004. Since 2004, they have seen a reduction of about 33 percent in the number of [natural and vitamin] products on store shelves.

Verkerk is bothered by the fact that the negative vitamin studies are so widely reported on by mainstream media while positive vitamin studies often receive no coverage.

> We have seen a lot of media bias, and all I can say is 'thank God for the Internet.' We are seeing clear censorship and even discrimination in the mainstream media. We have received five or six invitations during the past couple of years to sit down on television [BBC], usually during key time slots, to discuss issues, often with people who have a biased nature, such as mainstream doctors. In one hundred percent of the occasions during the last two or three years, they tell us at the very last minute that they are cancelling the program. In fact, we've been lied to and told that the program has been cancelled when it wasn't. In those cases, we were replaced with a pushover type of person. The researchers feel that we should be included, but at a higher level it is almost like we are blacklisted.

Media bias is not the only problem that Verkerk has had to deal with. "On a personal level, I had my house broken into and my computers taken. It wasn't broken into in a way in which a petty thief would break in. They are certainly very sophisticated break-ins," he said. Although the police were called and private investigators hired, the crime was never solved. "It doesn't dampen our resolve in any way," said Verkerk of the burglary. "I've spent twenty-five years of my life butting up against some of the biggest companies in the world in agriculture and health care. Inevitably, you do put a few people's noses out of joint."[45]

A Closer Look at DSHEA

The Dietary Supplement Health and Education Act protects dietary supplements from being regulated as drugs by the FDA. It appropriately classifies supplements and herbs as foods and does not limit their use. However, it also prevents dietary supplement manufacturers and food producers from making any health claims about their products. The act passed in response to a strong grassroots effort determined to keep the powerful pharmaceutical lobby from achieving its goal: to get dietary supplements classified as pharmaceuticals, which would have made therapeutic doses unavailable to consumers without a prescription. DSHEA protected supplements from FDA regulation with the exception of cases in which the FDA could prove a supplement wasn't safe. As a result, in the last 17 years, the dietary supplement industry has produced innovations that have benefitted millions of consumers who have used dietary supplements to improve their health.

However, in 2011, the FDA proposed new regulations that would undermine the protections provided by DSHEA and give the FDA authority to regulate "new dietary ingredients" introduced after October 15, 1994. As noted by the Alliance for Natural Health,[46] If the proposed regulations are implemented, some of the most effective nutrients available will be withdrawn from the market. These guidelines are so broad that the FDA can define almost anything as a "new" dietary ingredient. This means the following:

- If a supplement includes more of an ingredient than was used 17 years ago, even something like vitamin C, it's "new."
- If an ingredient uses a different extraction process, such as baking or fermentation, it's "new."

- If a supplement uses an ingredient at a different "life stage," such as using ripe rather than unripe apples, it's "new."

- If a supplement duplicates an ingredient in a laboratory rather than extracting it from the food—even though it's chemically identical—it's "new."

- If a probiotic formula includes a strain of bacteria that wasn't found in yogurt 17 years ago, it's "new."

As a result of these regulations, the manufacturers would have to take any "new" ingredients off the market until they could *prove* that the ingredients were safe—even if those ingredients have been safely used for 17 years.

The type of proof demanded by the FDA in this law would make it nearly impossible for manufacturers to comply. According to the guidelines, many companies would have to conduct one-year animal studies using a dosage that's *1,000 times* the typical dose. So, for instance, a fish oil manufacturer would have to conduct a one-year study where animals are force-fed the human equivalent of 240,000 mg of fish oil each and every day. This outrageous dose would injure the animals and give the FDA an excuse to outlaw the product. In addition, if one fish oil manufacturer performs a study that meets the FDA criteria, it doesn't mean the other fish oil makers can use the same data. Each manufacturer must do its own studies before it's allowed to sell its product.

These type of studies costs $100,000 to $200,000 for each ingredient. For those products that include multiple ingredients, it could cost millions of dollars for a company to get the products approved by the FDA. Few supplement makers will be able to afford these studies; many will be put out of business. Those companies that remain would still be at the mercy of the FDA. The FDA can approve or reject anything it wants for any reason. And in the past, it has rejected the majority of ingredients submitted to it. As a result, most of the nutrients that Americans buy today are at risk of being pulled from the market and never returning. Those that do return will be a lot more expensive or may be available only as prescription drugs.

The FDA's actions represent a blatant abuse of power. According to the law, the FDA has to prove a dietary supplement is unsafe for it to be taken off the market. These new guidelines ignore that requirement and are clearly not what congress intended.

The Dietary Supplement Labeling Act of 2011

At the same time that these regulatory guidelines were released, Senator Dick Durbin of Illinois introduced the Dietary Supplement Labeling Act of 2011 (S. 1310). Durbin's bill would allow the FDA to compile a list of all dietary ingredients it believed to have the potential for adverse health effects and require supplement manufacturers to add warning labels to any supplements containing those ingredients.

According to the very conservative *Washington Times,* this bill, combined with the FDA guidance on supplements,

> would force companies to pull these products off the shelves for months, if not for good, and significantly raise prices, making the remaining supplements expensive and harder to find. While it isn't a direct ban, regulatory hurdles such as these are a means by which government bureaucrats get in the way of individuals' ability to make their own decisions about their health care.[47]

The *Washington Times* further reported:

Many of the nutrients and minerals in supplements have been part of the human diet since the dawn of history and were used by doctors and in folk remedies for centuries. The supplements industry has a good record of safety, especially when compared with the FDA-regulated drug market. While there are some supplements with questionable benefits, the decision about which supplements are right for whom ought to be left to consumers and their medical care providers to determine.

The Durbin and FDA proposals do nothing to improve the safety of the supplement marketplace and likely will eliminate many of the available products. If the proposals are implemented, the increased cost and decreased variety will mean that many consumers, especially low-income ones, will be forced to stop taking the vitamins and nutrients that can benefit their long-term well-being. This unnecessary power grab would benefit FDA regulators and pharmaceutical companies by taking their competitors off the market, but it would harm the American public.[48]

According to The Alliance for Natural Health, "Government-mandated warnings on labels could say anything the government wants them to say, no matter how unreasonable, and could be of any length, even if the packaging became prohibitively expensive." The ANH is also concerned that the list of unsafe ingredients or doses would be based on completely arbitrary or nonexistent standards and that the FDA could, as a result, create completely unreasonable rules. In addition, the proposed rules include no process to challenge an FDA determination. The ANH also points out that the DSHEA already requires pre-preapproval of all health claims. Other laws already in place require adherence to good manufacturing practices and accurate disclosure of ingredients. All that Sen. Durbin's "Dietary Supplement Labeling Act" would do is make it more expensive to manufacture supplements, and it would discourage innovation.[49]

When Senator Durbin's bill was not referred out of committee for a vote after a few months, he and Senator Henry Waxman wrote a letter to the General Accounting Office (GAO) asking for a review of adverse event data, but only for supplements.

In response, The Alliance for Natural Health said :

> If consumer safety is really Sen. Durbin's motivation . . . why aren't he and Rep. Waxman also asking the GAO to review adverse event report (AER) data for vaccines and drugs, which are far more dangerous and have far more reported adverse events? Just look at the number of adverse events reported for 2008 alone:
>
> • Supplements: 1,080 adverse events[50], of which 672 were considered serious;
> • Vaccines: 26,517 adverse events[51], of which 3,923 were considered serious; and
> • Prescription drugs and "therapeutic biologics": 526,527 adverse events[52], of which 275,421 had serious outcomes."[53]

Even though these statistics show very dramatic differences in the safety profile of supplements versus pharmaceuticals, they don't tell the whole story. If the FDA-approved drug label states that it can cause fainting or nausea or chest pains or seizures, those side effects are considered to be within the range of expected outcomes and may not be reported.[54] At the same time, as *USA Today* reported, the FDA considers an adverse event related to a supplement to be "anything from a concern that a supplement isn't working to a serious illness that follows consumption"[55] that may or may not be causally related to the supplement.

The European Attempts to Restrict Use of Vitamins and Herbs

Attempts to restrict the availability of supplements and legal challenges to those restrictions have been playing out in the European Union for the last decade. It is only because of legal challenges and advocacy by natural medicine proponents that most supplements have remained on the market.

The European Union's Food Supplements Directive (FSD), the first Europeanwide legislation for food supplements, was adopted by the European Parliament and Council in 2002. It requires that all food supplements be proven safe in both dosage and purity. Food supplements are defined as being concentrated sources of nutrients or other substances with a nutritional or physiological effect whose purpose is to supplement the normal diet. In the United States, food supplements are generally referred to as vitamins and minerals.

Before the FSD was enacted, supplements were regulated differently by each of the 27 different countries that make up the European Union. Some supplements were regulated as food and others as medicine. Members of the European Union are required to follow the FSD because EU legislation takes precedence over the domestic legislation of each country.

The stated intention of the FSD is to protect the consumer from unsafe products and to prevent food supplements from being represented as medicine. The FSD dictates the maximum dosage levels for vitamins and minerals and sets rules for the labeling and advertising of food supplements. It establishes what is called a "positive list" for vitamins and minerals and required that all products not on the positive list be removed from store shelves by December 31, 2009. The positive list initially encompassed 28 vitamins and minerals (for example, vitamins A, D, E, and C; calcium; and magnesium) and 112 synthetic forms of these vitamins and minerals (for example, calcium carbonate, magnesium chloride, and retinol). Additional substances have been added to the positive list since the FSD was released in 2002; they now number 181.

Verkerk has responded to the FSD requirements:

> Because of the FSD's lack of clarity and restrictive interpretation by regulators, it was widely understood that to get an ingredient onto the positive list, manufacturers would have to go through a very time-consuming, onerous, and costly process for them to prove that each nutrient was safe. This might have cost more than £250,000 (over $300,000) per ingredient. With many innovative, leading-edge supplements containing sometimes upwards of 30 ingredients each, this burden upon many leading-edge manufacturers, typically being small companies, would effectively lead to them being put out of business. This would be the case even if the products included natural sources of vitamins and minerals that had been part of the human diet for thousands of years.[56]

A regulatory assessment conducted by the UK government agreed with the ANH and said, "Any reduction in the range of products on the market would also reduce consumer choice. For products containing substances excluded from the 'positive lists' but which we currently consider safe, this reduction in choice appears unnecessary."[57]

The ANH is based in the United Kingdom and has been opposed to the FSD. It said, "The impact of this directive, if allowed to be implemented in its current form, will be to remove access to over 300 vitamin and mineral ingredients currently available to UK consumers which translates into over 5,000 products."[58]

In addition to reducing consumer choice, the ANH believes that the FSD will set maximum dosages levels at unreasonably low levels. As an example, it points out that the FSD's recommended maximum dosage level for beta-carotene is less than what is present in two carrots.

Because it believed that the FSD was illegal under European law, that it had no scientific justification, and that it unfairly restricted commerce, the ANH challenged it in the High Court of Justice of England and Wales. The United Kingdom's National Association of Health Stores and Health Food Manufacturers also filed their own challenge with the court, and both challenges were eventually joined.

Before their case was presented, Verkerk said:

> We have the firm support of many of the world's leading scientific and medical experts in nutrition. Based on the most recent results of international research, the evidence conclusively shows that the nutrients under threat of the ban are not only safe but also beneficial in promoting optimum health in many millions of people. Based upon the

premise of good science and good law this ban should be overturned.[59]

The April 5, 2005, opinion issued by the Advocate General of the High Court concluded that the FSD was invalid. It wrote:

> Examination of the provisions of Directive 2002/46/EC of the European Parliament and of the Council on the approximation of the laws of the Member States relating to food supplements has disclosed that the Directive infringes the principle of proportionality, because basic principles of Community law, such as the requirements of legal protection, of legal certainty and of sound administration have not been properly taken into account. The Directive is, therefore, invalid.[60]

In European law, the principle of proportionality requires each decision and measure to be based on a fair assessment and balancing of interests.[61]

The advocate general was also critical of the design of the FSD and said:

> In short, this procedure, in so far as it may exist and in so far as it may deserve this title, has the transparency of a black box: no provision is made for parties to be heard, no time-limits apply in respect of decision-making; nor, indeed, is there any certainty that a final decision will be taken. The procedure therefore lacks essential guarantees for the protection of the interests of private applicants.[62]

The opinion of the advocate general was strictly a legal opinion, and the final decision on the legal challenge had to be made by the European Court of Justice (ECJ) in Luxembourg. In the majority of cases, the ECJ upholds the advisory decisions of the advocate general. On July 12, 2005, the 13-judge panel of the ECJ concluded that the FSD did not infringe on the principal of proportionality. They voted unanimously to uphold the FSD.

Despite the ruling, the ANH considered it a victory. ANH issued a press release after the ruling that read:

> It is not a simple question of whether the FSD was lawful or not. The devil, as always, is in the details. ANH challenged the lawfulness of the FSD because to ANH it appeared to have draconian and quite unnecessary consequences for the food supplements industry and for consumers. In upholding the lawfulness of the FSD, the ECJ has clarified what exactly the FSD actually means and has clearly restricted the scope of the application of the ban on non-FSD compliant nutrients. There are very significant and positive details within the judgment that will be beneficial to the millions of consumers who use vitamin and mineral supplements for their health and are key to everything that ANH has been campaigning for all along.[63]

Because of the clarifications made during the ruling, the directive no longer applies to natural forms of vitamins and minerals normally found in the diet. A diverse variety of vitamins and minerals was determined to be outside the directive's scope and will therefore continue to be regulated as foods. The clarified interpretation of the directive also makes it much simpler, less time consuming, and more affordable for a vitamin or mineral to gain admission to the positive list. Because of the ruling, any refusal to add a product to the positive list can also be challenged in the courts. It also shifts a considerable amount of the burden of proof of safety away from the manufacturer and toward the regulator. The ruling implies that a ban cannot be implemented on a supplement unless a risk to public health following a scientific risk assessment can be proven. The European Food Safety Authority is the agency responsible for the scientific assessment of supplements.

According to Verkerk:

> The fact that the necessary requirements for admission to the positive list have been fundamentally changed now means that the vast majority of high-quality and innovative vitamin and mineral food supplements will now, with relative ease and limited expense, be able to join the positive list and thus not face a ban. These changes to the positive list have been at the heart of what the ANH has been campaigning for over the last three and a half years and, indeed, formed the major part of its legal challenge to aspects of the Food Supplements Directive. In achieving this, ANH has therefore gained a very significant victory for consumers, practitioners, retailers and manufacturers in protecting their right to buy, supply and produce safe, innovative and leading-edge food supplements across Europe.[64]

Despite the victories, Verkerk points out that some supplements have been banned from the market in the EU. Many mineral amino acid chelates and all mineral orotates, ketoglutarates, and products containing vanadium and silver are among the banned supplements.

Although the FSD has not caused the feared increases in supplement costs, it has caused problems for smaller retailers. Again, according to Verkerk:

> The positive list has meant that major multiples [supermarkets] are taking share away from smaller specialist retailers [independent health stores] given that it is difficult for the latter to compete on price. The dramatic decline in diversity of products resulting from a narrow positive list system creates a "me too" environment in which large corporations are able to exploit their low raw material costs—drug companies are still by far the largest producer of raw materials for vitamin, mineral and amino acid based products—their economies of scale and of course their well-greased international distribution networks.

The ANH continues to work on other issues related to the use of supplements in the EU. It is concerned about legislation that could restrict the maximum permitted dosage levels of vitamins and minerals. Says Verkerk:

> The European Commission proposal on this has still not been forthcoming, this being down to a number of factors including the fact that we have maintained

petitions in the European Parliament that are critical of the scientific methods being used to determine maximum levels. We have also published two major scientific papers in a leading peer-reviewed scientific journal critiquing these methods.

The ANH is also concerned with regulations directed at the health claims that appear on the labels of foods and food supplements. The European Food Safety Authority (EFSA) has spent several years evaluating these health claims. According to the EFSA:

Since 2008 the Panel has assessed 2,758 food-related general function health claims to determine whether they were supported by sound scientific evidence, thereby assisting the European Commission and Member States in establishing a list of cla

Verkerk believes in truth in labeling but says:

Once this list is passed into law, around two thousand five hundred commonly used claims about the health benefits of foods and food ingredients (health claims) will be banned. In the past, these health claims are likely to have made it easier for you to choose particular foods and food supplements to help manage your own health or that of friends or family. By comparison, the marketplace used by future generations will contain only a very limited number of frequently repeated, generalized health claims. With such limited information available, it will be much harder to choose foods and natural health products based on their specific health benefits. The passage of the general function health claims list is undergoing scrutiny in the European Parliament, and we are trying to achieve a veto of the proposal because, while it will legitimize just two hundred and twenty heath claims on commercial food and natural health products, it will simultaneously ban more than two thousand five hundred.

The Threat from Codex

An international effort known as the Codex Alimentarius Commission (generally referred to as Codex) is also threatening consumer access to nutritional supplements and has met with success in some European countries. Codex was established in 1961 by the Food and Agriculture Organization of the United Nations (FAO) and was joined, in 1962, by the World Health Organization (WHO). The commission's main goals are to protect consumer health and ensure fair practices in the international food trade. The Codex Alimentarius is recognized by WHO as an international reference point for the resolution of disputes concerning food safety and consumer protection. Today, however, Codex is spearheaded by the pharmaceutical companies and seeks to criminalize the possession of nonprescribed vitamins in dosages greater than the recommended daily allowance. Codex classifies supplements as toxins, which must be regulated to protect consumers.

Currently, DSHEA protects the United States from Codex's vitamin and mineral guidelines. The strength and monetary power of those lobbying Congress on behalf of Codex, however, are sufficient to turn this around. By projecting false information that nutrients are toxins, it generates calls to "protect" people from these substances. The next step would be the setting of ultralow permissible dosages of supplements. If Codex is implemented in the United States, therapeutic dosages of vitamins and minerals will become unavailable and, in fact, illegal. Only intentionally ineffective, ultralow dose supplements would be legal. Nutritional supplement manufacturers and health food stores would likely go out of business. Natural health practitioners would lose the tools of their trade and Americans would lose their opportunity to choose to treat themselves with natural options. The only winner would be "big pharma."

One Final Threat from Home

Further threatening the use of dietary supplements is an ongoing effort by the American Dietetic Association to pass legislation that would prohibit anyone except registered dieticians from talking to patients about nutrition—even physicians trained in nutrition. Most dieticians do not receive training in using supplements to treat diseases. Generally, they are trained in nutrient and diet management as well as in institutional food service. For example, dieticians are responsible for designing balanced and special diet meals for populations in hospitals, schools, and nursing homes. They are generally against the use of supplements because they believe that all nutritional needs can be met with a balanced diet. This claim has been proven false in thousands of studies.

Food Sensitivities and Toxins

Pain can also be caused by food sensitivities and reactions to toxins in food. Two examples are gluten sensitivity—including the more severe form, celiac disease—and reactions to aspartame (NutraSweet), a neurotoxin.

Gluten

According to the National Foundation for Celiac Awareness, celiac disease is an autoimmune disease triggered by eating gluten, a protein found in wheat, barley, and rye. When a person with celiac disease eats a food containing gluten, the immune system attacks finger-like structures in the small intestine called the villi. Damaged villi in turn interfere with the body's ability to absorb nutrients, and malnutrition can occur. This can lead to other serious complications, including other autoimmune diseases, osteoporosis, cancer, and thyroid disease.[65] It's estimated that 3 million Americans have celiac disease and that most cases are undiagnosed.

More than 300 symptoms of celiac disease have been identified. The mix of symptoms varies from person to person. Some may have gastrointestinal symptoms; others, irritability, depression, joint pain, tingling, numbness, or fatigue. Some people develop symptoms in childhood; others feel healthy until they are much older.[66]

It's estimated that 18 million Americans have nonceliac gluten sensitivity. Individuals with this disorder have gluten intolerance and experience celiac disease-like symptoms but don't experience the intestinal damage found in celiac disease. Recent research indicates that the immune system mechanisms of the two disorders are different and that gluten sensitivity is a less severe disorder than celiac disease. Both disorders improve with avoidance of gluten.[67]

Tony

As a child, Tony experienced joint pain that doctors were unable to diagnose. The pain began to intensify when he was in his 30s. By the time he was 36, the pain in his arms, hands, and feet had become so severe that he knew that it was time to see a doctor. According to Tony, the doctor took one look at him and told him that he could solve his pain problems if he lost weight. Tony is 6'7" tall. At the time, he competed in strongmen competitions and, despite weighing 400 pounds, had only 10% body fat. He followed the advice of his doctor and lost 70 pounds. The pain only got worse.

"I went back to the doctor, and he told me that I was still too heavy and that I needed to lose more weight," remembered Tony.

Once again, he followed doctor's orders and dropped another 60 pounds. Tony couldn't believe it when the doctor told him that he was still too heavy. He now weighed 270 pounds and had only 20 pounds of fat on his entire body.

In addition to telling Tony to lose weight, the doctor ran a variety of tests to rule out vascular and heart problems. When the tests came back normal and the weight loss did not affect his joint pain, Tony was prescribed narcotic pain pills for his symptoms. Because he is a police officer, Tony was unable to take these drugs. He resigned himself to living in pain.

A short time later, Tony slipped a disc in his back while on the job.

Tony (cont.)

Because his workers' compensation doctors just prescribed more pain pills, he sought help for the injury from an acupuncturist. The acupuncturist gave him a physical before treating his back and diagnosed Tony with celiac disease. He told him to eliminate gluten from his diet and to see if that had any effect on his joint pain. "Two days later, I was pain free," said Tony. None of the doctors had ever tested him for celiac disease.

If celiac disease is suspected, it can be easily diagnosed through blood tests and intestinal biopsies.

Acupuncturists are often able to make the celiac diagnosis based entirely on a physical examination. According to Dr. John Stump, diagnosis is based on irregularities in the pulse, coating on the tongue, appearance of the eye, and tender points on the ear.[68]

Today, Tony continues his gluten-free diet. His joint pain never returned. He believes that his doctors were too quick to blame his problems on his size. He also believes that they should have continued to look for the source of his problems before prescribing pills to mask the pain.

Janice

Janice, one of my clients, came to her first session with me in a great deal of emotional distress. She reported that she had been in a severe state of emotional turmoil for the last eight years. Her extreme distress started when her son overdosed and almost died, and her current husband, her son's stepfather, had failed to immediately come to her aid. Given her protracted negative state of mind, I was very surprised to see on her intake form that she was in remission from rheumatoid arthritis. When I asked her about it, she told me that she cut gluten out of her diet and the problem resolved. If she had not made this dietary change before coming to me and still had active arthritis symptoms when we met, I would have assumed that the problem was related to her emotional state and not her diet.

Aspartame

Aspartame (brand names NutraSweet and Equal) is a synthetic calorie-free sweetener used in more than 90 countries in more than 6,000 products.[69] A 2007 comprehensive review of the published literature in a toxicology journal concluded that there is no evidence to support any connection between aspartame and problems with nervous system function, learning, behavior, or cancer.[70] Numerous individuals, however, have reported that while ingesting aspartame they developed neurological symptoms, including chronic pain, and that within days of stopping use of aspartame their pain disappeared. For those who tried reintroducing aspartame, the pain returned, according to the Aspartame Toxicity Information Center.[71]

Mary

Mary, one of my clients who suffered from severe joint pain, confessed to drinking diet soda "all day long." When I mentioned the possibility of a pain–aspartame connection, she switched to unsweetened ice tea. Within a few days, she was pain free. She was able to stop her pain medication, which had a side effect of interfering with fertility. She had been going through fertility treatments unsuccessfully and had stopped trying. Within a short time of stopping her pain medication, she became pregnant.

Most people who consume artificial sweeteners do so because they believe it will help them lose weight or at least avoid gaining weight. However, people who consume artificial sweeteners tend to gain more weight than people who do not, according to a 2010 Yale review of available studies.[72]

My Diet Soda Addiction

I was a diet soda addict for most of my life. The idea that I could, as I saw it, "get something for nothing" (consume sweet beverages and foods without the added calories) kept me hooked for decades. Then a nutritionist told me that artificial sweeteners actually make people fatter because their bodies interpret the sweet taste as a need for insulin to process it. The insulin lowers blood sugar, leading to increased hunger. That information finally convinced me to stop consuming artificial sweeteners. Though I personally did not notice any changes in terms of susceptibility to pain, I am currently slimmer than I was when consuming artificial sweeteners.

So, if you are in chronic pain and use artificial sweeteners, it's probably a good idea to curtail your use.

Tobacco

Smoking tobacco increases the risk of low-back pain and degenerative changes in the spine, according to many studies. Chemicals found in tobacco may reduce the blood supply to nerves, muscles, and other soft tissue, making injury more likely and healing more difficult.[73]

Other Allergens and Toxins That Can Cause Pain

A comprehensive review of all the allergens and toxins that can cause pain is beyond the scope of this book. Be aware, however, that many commonly found substances can cause or exacerbate your pain. This issue is worth investigating. MSG, a common flavor enhancer found in most processed foods, is another likely culprit.

Chapter 8

HERBAL TREATMENTS

There is fossil evidence of humans using plants as medicine as long as 60,000 years ago.[1] Although botanical medicine is considered alternative medicine in Western societies, it is the dominant form of medicine in a large part of the world, including China, India, and parts of South America and Africa.[2] The World Health Organization estimates that 80% of the world's population uses herbal medicine for at least some part of their primary health care. Many herbs are recognized as effective for the treatment of various medical conditions by authoritative sources, including the World Health Organization, the European Scientific Cooperative on Phytomedicine, and the German Commission E.[3]

Most modern pharmaceuticals are derived from plants. Pharmacologists look to nature for plants known in traditional cultures to promote desired biological activity. Then they identify and isolate an active ingredient to study its chemical structure. This ingredient may become a drug, or the chemical structure may be modified to make a more potent drug. However, drugs derived from an isolated component of a plant tend to be more toxic, and to have more side effects, than the original herb. This is because whole plants have other ingredients that protect our bodies from potential negative effects. Clinical benefits of herbs are also superior because the natural material has many other components that support healing via similar or related pathways.[4]

Many herbs have not been submitted to what is considered the "gold standard" of Western medicine—the double-blinded randomized controlled study. However, their traditional uses are the result of hundreds or thousands of years of trial and error and observations by indigenous healers, often across many geographic regions if the plant is widely available. Is this really a less stringent test than a test of a pharmaceutical that is conducted for four to eight weeks on a limited population by a company that serves to benefit substantially if it can "prove" its drug has positive effects?

Herbs useful in pain management include those that have analgesic, anti-inflammatory, antispasmodic, detoxifying, or sedative effects. Multiple herbs can be combined to address different aspects of a pain problem.[5]

The *PDR for Herbal Medicines* is modeled after the *Physician's Desk Reference (PDR) for Prescription Drugs*. It reviews 700 of the most commonly used herbal remedies, their indications and usage, clinical study results where available, and possible interactions with prescription drugs.[6] The *PDR for Herbal Medicines* lists 121 herbs with analgesic effects, 24 with anti-inflammatory effects, 38 with sedative/hypnotic effects, 36 with antispasmodic effects, and 22 that have been used to treat migraines.

An exhaustive review of herbs useful in the treatment of pain is beyond the scope of this book, but I will describe a few herbs that are helpful in decreasing pain. Where there have been clinical studies, I will cite them.

One of the most potent botanicals for the treatment of pain is cannabis, also known as marijuana. Marijuana is both unique and uniquely controversial, so it has its own chapter in this book.

Some Herbs That Are Useful for Pain

Boswellia

Frankincense, an extract from the Boswellia (Boswellia sacra or serrata) species of trees, has been used medicinally for thousands of years. Currently grown in India, Africa, China, and the Middle East, it is most commonly used for the treatment of inflammatory diseases, including asthma, arthritis, chronic pain syndrome, chronic bowel diseases, and cancer.[7] There is now research evidence to support all of those uses. Studies have also found that frankincense improves learning and memory.[8]

Research has shown that Boswellia inhibits leukotrienes, chemicals produced by the body that can cause inflammation by promoting free-radical damage, autoimmune responses, migration of inflammation-causing cells to the area of inflammation, and cell adhesion. Diseases caused by leukotrienes include arthritis, rheumatism, colitis, psoriasis, and asthma. Boswellia shrinks inflamed tissue and is nontoxic.[9]

Two double-blind randomized placebo-controlled studies of patients with osteoarthritis of the knee found that Boswellia extracts decreased pain, improved function, and improved the condition of the knee joint. Some patients started feeling better in as few as seven days after starting treatment.[10,11]

Boswellia extracts have also been shown to be effective in the treatment of inflammatory bowel diseases. Two studies of patients with ulcerative colitis found significant improvements: 82% of the Boswellia-treated patients went into remission in one study[12] and 70% in another study.[13] In both studies, the Boswellia extracts outperformed the standard drug treatment regimen.

Osteopathic physician E.W. McDonagh reported that he has treated hundreds of patients with Boswellia for a wide variety of chronic musculoskeletal conditions, including arthritis, muscle pain, degenerative joint disease, muscle wasting, and sciatic pain. He reported that within two to four weeks, all of his patients experienced substantial reductions in pain and were able to significantly reduce or eliminate their other medications.[14]

Butterbur

Butterbur (Petasites hybridus) is an herb native to Europe, Southwest Asia, and North Africa. Butterbur has been used medicinally for more than 2,000 years to treat allergies, asthma, headache, and muscle spasms. A butterbur root extract has been available by prescription in Germany since 1988.[15]

The American Academy of Neurology, in a 2012 evidence-based guideline update of NSAIDs and other complementary treatments for migraine prevention, listed butterbur as the only treatment with "established efficacy" for migraine prevention.[16] This classification was based on two scientifically rigorous studies. In one randomized double-blind placebo-controlled study, migraine headache frequency was reduced by up to 60% with twice daily doses of 50 mg of Petasites hybridus extract, with no reported adverse effects.[17] In a second randomized study, which compared 75 mg twice daily of Petasites hybridus with 50 mg twice daily and placebo, headache frequency was reduced 48% for the 75 mg group, 36% for the 50 mg group, and 26% for the placebo group. The only adverse effect reported in some patients was burping.[18] The American Academy of Neurology guideline states that butterbur "should be offered" to migraine patients.[19]

In my 22-plus years of treating migraine patients, I have reviewed many lists of doctor-prescribed medications and supplements. I have never seen butterbur listed.

Cat's Claw

Cat's claw (Uncaria tomentosa and Uncaria guianensis) is a vine found in the basin of the Amazon River and has anti-inflammatory properties. The bark is traditionally used in South America to treat arthritis, bursitis, lupus, chronic fatigue syndrome, and stomach and intestinal disorders.[20]

A four-week study in 2001 comparing cat's claw to placebo in patients with osteoarthritis of the knee found that pain associated with activity was significantly reduced. Improvement was found within the first week of therapy. Knee pain at night and at rest was not improved during the brief study period. There were no significant side effects.[21]

A 2007 study compared a combination herbal supplement, Reparagen, and glucosamine sulfate (see description following) in the treatment of mild to moderate knee osteoarthritis. Reparagen combines cat's claw with an extract of a South American vegetable, Lepidium meyenii, in the Cruciferous family. This eight-week randomized double-blind controlled study found that both supplements reduced pain by 60% in eight weeks. Both reduced stiffness by eight weeks, glucosamine by 61% and Reparagen by 51%. Use of acetaminophen was less in the Reparagen group. Improvements were seen within the first week of treatment, and improvements increased over the course of the study.[22]

A 24-week randomized double-blind placebo-controlled study in 2002 evaluated cat's claw for treatment of rheumatoid arthritis. Patients receiving cat's claw had a 53.2% reduction in painful joints compared to 24.1% in the placebo group.[23]

Feverfew

Feverfew (Chrysanthemum parthenium) is most frequently used to prevent migraine headaches. It has also been traditionally used for fever, stiffness, skin conditions, and gynecological disorders. The American Academy of Neurology, in a 2012 evidence-based guideline update, listed feverfew as "probably effective" for migraine prevention.[24]

In one randomized placebo-controlled double-blind study of feverfew, migraines decreased from 4.76 to 2.86 headaches per month, a decrease of 1.9 attacks/month, compared to a decrease of 1.3 attacks in the placebo group.[25]

Warning: Don't suddenly stop taking feverfew, because you may experience withdrawal symptoms, including rebound headaches, anxiety, sleep disturbances, muscle stiffness, and muscle pain. Avoid taking if pregnant; it may cause a miscarriage. Feverfew may also reduce the effectiveness of antidepressant drugs.[26]

Ginger

Ginger (Zingiber officinale) is native to India and is also grown in Asia, Africa, Latin America, and Australia. Ginger has been used medicinally in China and India for more than 2,500 years for many conditions, including headaches, arthritis, nausea, and vomiting. It has also been used as an antimicrobial and antifungal agent.[27]

A 2015 review and meta-analysis of five randomized controlled trials of the use of ginger for the treatment of osteoarthritis found that ginger significantly reduced pain and disability compared to treatment with a placebo.[28] Another 2015 literature review and meta-analysis of randomized double-blinded placebo-controlled trials of ginger and turmeric (a related compound) for the treatment of pain found that the herbs were clinically effective in reducing subjective chronic pain and that they were safer than NSAIDs. Significant positive effects were found for arthritis, primary dysmenorrhea, pain recovery from surgery, and pain from delayed onset muscle soreness. The review also found that the higher the dose, the larger the reduction in pain.

One safety issue identified was that both NSAIDs and ginger extracts were associated with a heightened bleeding risk, though the comparative risk has never been studied.[29]

Green Tea

Tea is a popular beverage all over the world. Compounds found in green tea (Camellia sinensis), especially epigallocatechin-3-gallate (EGCG), have been found to have anticancer, antidiabetic, anti-inflammatory, antibacterial, antiobesity, and neuro-protective effects. Numerous studies have shown that EGCG inhibits inflammation and other biochemical precursors to osteoarthritis.[30] Green tea consumption is considered not only safe but also health promoting.[31]

Curcumin

Curcumin (curcuma longa, also known as turmeric), an herb with anti-inflammatory effects, is native to southwest India. It is used as a spice and is the ingredient that gives curry and mustards their yellow color. It has been used medicinally in India for thousands of years to treat diseases of the skin, pulmonary and gastrointestinal systems, aches, pains, wounds, sprains, and liver disorders.[32] Curcumin has been shown to have antioxidant, anti-inflammatory, antiviral, antibacterial, antifungal, and anticancer effects.[33] Interest has recently been growing in studying its medicinal effects.

A small randomized eight-week study in 2012 of 45 patients in India with rheumatoid arthritis compared the safety and effectiveness of curcumin alone, diclofenac sodium (Voltaren, a NSAID) alone, and the two in combination. All three groups significantly improved in measures of disease severity. But the curcumin group did the best in terms of pain severity, total number of painful joints, total swollen joints, patients' global assessment of functioning, and physicians' global assessment of functioning. The curcumin alone group did better than the combination group. There were no adverse effects from the curcumin.[34]

A 2014 randomized controlled study in Thailand compared the effectiveness and safety of curcumin and ibuprofen in 367 patients with knee osteoarthritis over a four-week period. The study found that curcumin was as effective as ibuprofen for relieving symptoms, with fewer gastrointestinal side effects.[35]

Preliminary studies in mice have shown that curcumin can reduce diabetic neuropathy pain.[36] Curcumin has also been shown to reduce postsurgical pain.[37]

Glucosamine and Chondroitin Sulphate

Glucosamine and chondroitin sulfate are natural substances normally found in joint cartilage. They have been used medicinally in supplements in Europe and Asia for more than 40 years.[38] Glucosamine is a type of sugar believed to be important in the formation and repair of cartilage. Chondroitin is part of a protein called proteoglycan, which is responsible for the elasticity of cartilage.[39] Numerous studies have been conducted on these supplements, alone and in combination.

The first two double-blind placebo-controlled randomized controlled trials using glucosamine and chondroitin sulfate for knee osteoarthritis, published in 1998, showed significant clinical improvement in symptoms.[40,41]

The most publicized study of these supplements was the Glucosamine/Chondroitin Arthritis Intervention Trial (GAIT), published in 2006 in the *New England Journal of Medicine*. The study included 1,583 osteoarthritis patients randomly assigned to receive either 1500 mg glucosamine, 1200 mg chondroitin, both glucosamine and chondroitin, 200 mg of celecoxib (a prescription drug, brand name Celebrex), or a placebo for 24 weeks. The glucosamine used was glucosamine hydrochloride rather than the glucosamine sulfate used in most supplements. Most patients had mild pain; 79 had moderate to severe pain. The results: 60% of the placebo group had a clinically meaningful improvement. Celecoxib was statistically significantly better than placebo in the mild pain group but not in the moderate to severe group. Glucosamine and chondroitin did not perform better than placebo in the mild pain group, but were significantly better than either placebo or celecoxib in the group with moderate to severe pain.[42]

The way the GAIT study was reported in the media made it appear that glucosamine and chondroitin did not work. For instance, the headline reporting on the study in the *New York Times* was, "Supplements Fail to Stop Arthritis Pain, Study Said."[43] Only if readers read the entire article would they would find out that it performed significantly better than the placebo and the prescription drug for those with the most severe pain. The authors of the GAIT study had financial relationships with Pfizer, the company that manufactures celecoxib.[44]

A 2009 meta-analyses of studies of glucosamine and chondroitin concluded that the supplements are safe and helpful in treating the symptoms of osteoarthritis. The review also reported that the supplements seem to have disease-modifying effects.[45]

In a 2014 Australian study known as the LEGS (Long-term Evaluation of Glucosamine Sulfate) study, patients received glucosamine 1500 mg per day, chondroitin 800 mg per day, both supplements, or a placebo for a period of two years. There was a clinically significant difference in the combination supplement group in joint space narrowing that study investigators believed was positive and clinically meaningful. All of the active treatment groups also showed improvements in pain over the course of the study. But none of the differences was statistically significant compared to the placebo group.[46]

In 2015, the MOVES six-month study also showed positive results. The study was conducted in Europe, where glucosamine and chondroitin are offered together as a prescription drug. The drug, Droglican, contains 500 mg glucosamine and 400 mg chondroitin and is taken three times daily. The study compared Droglican with celecoxib in patients with moderate to severe osteoarthritis pain. Both groups had similar reductions in pain, stiffness, swelling, mobility, self-care, and depression. The study investigators considered glucosamine and chondroitin the superior treatment because, unlike celecoxib, the supplements alter the underlying disease process, and because they do not pose the cardiovascular and gastrointestinal risks of celecoxib.[47]

A 2005 study conducted in Belgium evaluated the use of a combination supplement containing glucosamine sulfate for low-back pain. The supplement also contained a botanical extract containing phytonutrients with anti-inflammatory properties and methylsulfonyl-methane (MSM), a sulfur found in fruits and vegetables. The 12-week study compared a group receiving conventional treatment only (physical therapy plus analgesics/anti-inflammatories) to a group that received conventional treatment plus the supplement. By the fourth week, the group taking the supplement had significantly greater improvements in pain at rest and lower back stiffness than the control group. Quality of life was also improved in the glucosamine group compared to the control group, but the difference was not statistically significant.[48]

For best results, both supplements should be taken together. Studies testing glucosamine and chondroitin individually have shown inconsistent results.[49] It is also important to buy these supplements from a reputable manufacturer, as some studies have shown that some brands don't contain much glucosamine or chondroitin.

CHAPTER 9
EXERCISE

Until almost the end of the 20th century, the conventional medical community recommended prolonged bed rest for back pain. It's only recently that physicians have begun recognizing that inactivity leads to weakness and deconditioning that can exacerbate pain problems.[1] Each day of bed rest can result in a loss of 1% to 3% of muscle strength. Muscles will also stiffen. The only cure is appropriate exercise.[2]

Muscles can also be the primary cause of pain. Common causes of muscle pain are muscle tension, weakness, stiffness, spasm, and trigger points.[3]

Muscle spasms, which come on quickly and can be excruciating, can result from unaccustomed exercise or other activities. They often go away themselves over time or can be broken up by using heat or ice and then gently stretching the involved muscle.[4]

Muscle weakness and stiffness occur when we don't get enough of the proper kind of exercise. This is also referred to as deconditioning. Exercise should begin with relaxation, to ease any tension in the muscle, and should then involve moving the muscle being exercised through its range of movement (limbering) followed by gentle stretching to overcome stiffness before attempting to strengthen the muscle. Healthy muscles not only are strong but also have a good range of motion, or flexibility. Exercising without stretching can create stiff muscles, which are more easily injured. It can be harder to overcome stiffness than weakness. Couch potatoes have both weakness and stiffness and are especially ripe for injury.[5] If we don't put our muscles through a full range of motion, they become stiff in the areas where they rarely or never move.[6]

Another way that muscles can contribute to pain is that when we are already in pain, we change the way we stand, sit, move, and lift to place less stress on the painful area. Over time, these unnatural changes to posture and movement may produce more soft tissue imbalances and pain.[7]

Many people in chronic pain avoid exercise because they are afraid of further injury and pain. Avoiding activity because of fear of pain is called kinesiophobia.[8]

The Kraus-Weber Exercises

In the early 1940s, Dr. Sonja Weber and Dr. Hans Kraus developed the Kraus-Weber test for minimum muscular strength and flexibility while working at Columbia Presbyterian Hospital in New York City. These tests require patients to perform simple exercises that test the strength of the upper and lower abdominal, psoas (hip flexor), and upper and lower back muscles as well as flexibility of the hamstrings. In a 1946 study Weber and Kraus conducted of 3,000 people with back pain, they found that only 18% had pathology that explained the pain. The other 82%, who had no identifiable pathology for their back pain, did fail at least one of the six Kraus-Weber tests.[9] These tests, along with the Kraus-Weber corrective exercises, are described in detail in Dr. Norman Marcus's book *End Back Pain Forever: A Groundbreaking Approach to Eliminating Your Suffering*.[10]

In 2001, a US review of published literature on 20,000 patients with low-back pain found that sprains and strains of muscles, tendons, and ligaments (collectively known as soft tissue) caused 70% to 80% of all low-back pain.[11]

Many other pain conditions are related to soft tissue abnormalities. Recent studies have shown that the muscles in patients diagnosed with fibromyalgia can be the most significant cause of pain. Muscles can also be a significant source of pain in patients with rheumatoid arthritis and osteoarthritis.[12]

For decades now, conventional medicine has relied on X-rays, MRIs, and CT scans to diagnose pain problems. However, none of this high-tech imagery can detect soft tissue abnormalities, which might be the cause of pain.[13] The only way to determine whether soft tissue is a source of pain is by manual physical examination.[14]

John F. Kennedy

President John F. Kennedy suffered from severe back pain when he came to the White House. Before becoming president, he had already experienced two failed back surgeries, the first when he was 27 years old. Kennedy's back pain was so severe at one point that he sometimes used crutches. His Secret Service agents were worried that he would end up in a wheelchair. Dr. Hans Kraus, called in to treat him in October 1961, found that Kennedy's back muscles were weak and stiff, his abdominal muscles atrophied, and his leg muscles extremely tight. Within a month of doing the prescribed Kraus-Weber exercises, Kennedy's strength and flexibility had improved and his back pain had significantly decreased. He was able, for the first time, to pick up his then two-year-old son, John.[15]

From 1976 to 1988, more than 300,000 people around the world, including in the United States, participated in the "Y's Way to a Healthy Back," a six-week program offered at YMCAs that was based on the Kraus-Weber exercises.[16] I was one of them. The program was extremely valuable in helping me to recover from my deconditioned state, which resulted from three years of inactivity because of severe back pain and fear of reinjury. The most comprehensive study of the YMCA program included 11,809 participants and found that after six weeks of the program, 81% reported no pain or reduced pain. 83% of the 546 participants who had pain after back surgery reported less pain. Those participants who best adhered to the program and had the most measured improvement in strength and flexibility had the largest decreases in pain.[17] Unfortunately, the YMCA discontinued the program after Alexander Melleby, the physical educator who had brought the program into the YMCA, retired.[18]

The muscles in the abdomen, back, and pelvis, collectively known as core muscles, stabilize the pelvis and spine. When they are weak, low-back pain can occur. Pilates exercise is effective for correcting this problem, as are the Kraus-Weber exercises.[19]

More Research Results

A 2005 systematic review of exercise therapy for chronic low-back pain concluded that individually designed, supervised exercise programs that include stretching or strengthening may improve pain and function in chronic nonspecific low-back pain.[20]

Exercise has also been shown effective for chronic neck pain. A 2014 review of available research on physical therapy interventions concluded that active strengthening exercises increased strength, improved function, reduced pain, and improved health-related quality of life. Adding stretching and aerobic exercise to treatment enhanced all of these benefits.[21] Exercise significantly reduced pain in both the short and intermediate term in a 2013 review of therapeutic exercise for chronic neck pain.[22]

Twelve weeks of aerobic exercise of moderate intensity improved physical function and overall well-being of those with fibromyalgia, but it was less effective in reducing pain or tender points, according to a 2008 Cochrane review of published research. Strength training for 12 weeks resulted in large reductions in pain, tender points, and depression as well as large improvements in overall well-being but was less effective in improving physical function.[23] It seems reasonable to conclude that an exercise program that combines aerobic exercise and strength training would improve all aspects of fibromyalgia.

Dr. Winfried Hauser, a German MD and researcher who has published extensively on fibromyalgia, stated at a 2013 international scientific meeting in Paris, "Aerobic exercise is the most effective weapon we have" for patients with fibromyalgia.[24]

For rheumatoid arthritis, it has been found that aerobic exercise and strengthening programs are effective and safe, according to a 2006 review of studies. The exercise programs reduced bone mineral loss and reduced joint damage.[25]

A 2013 meta-analysis of exercise interventions for lower limb osteoarthritis (knee and hip) found that exercise interventions significantly improve pain and function. The most effective interventions were found to be those that combined strengthening exercises with exercises that improved flexibility and aerobic capacity, either on land or in water.[26]

Even though arthritis is a disease of the joints, strengthening the muscles helps because muscles act as "shock absorbers" in the body, lessening the impact of movement on arthritic joints. The exercises must be intense enough to significantly improve muscle strength to be effective.[27]

A 2014 study followed 1,788 adults with or at risk of knee osteoarthritis over a two-year period and found that those who walked more had better function. Walking more than 6,000 steps a day protected against developing functional limitations, and each additional 1,000 steps a day resulted in a 16% to 18% reduction in problems in function.[28]

Exercise doesn't have to be structured to aid in alleviating pain and improving function. A recent study of sedentary patients with chronic low-back pain compared a six-week aerobic treadmill walking program to a program of specific back muscle strengthening exercises. The study found that both types of exercise were equally effective in improving function in people with chronic low-back pain.[29]

Aquatic Exercise

Exercising in water can also be very beneficial in the alleviation of pain and may enable patients with significant mobility issues to exercise. Water immersion for physical rehabilitation and spiritual renewal has been practiced throughout the world since ancient times.[30] In modern times, during the polio epidemics of the 1900s, active movement was added to water therapy.[31] Water's property of buoyancy reduces pressure on joints, decreasing pain and making movement easier. The effective body weight in neck-deep water is only about 10% of the total on land; in chest deep immersion, it's 25%. This makes it easier for pain patients to engage in exercise and to strengthen joint-supporting muscles. Warm water immersion also relaxes muscles and may help the body eliminate pain-inducing toxins from soft tissue.[32]

Franklin D. Roosevelt

President Franklin D. Roosevelt was an avid proponent of water therapy. He suffered from partial paralysis as a result of contracting polio when he was 39 years old. A friend recommended to FDR that he visit a resort in Warm Springs, Georgia, to bathe in its warm mineral-rich waters. He was thrilled to discover the water was so buoyant that he could walk around in it without his braces. In 1927, he purchased the property and transformed it into a treatment center for polio patients. Thousands of polio victims have gone there for treatment over the years.[33]

A 12-week study of fibromyalgia patients and warm water immersion, with and without exercise, found that both groups obtained significant and similar relief from most fibromyalgia symptoms, but the group that exercised had longer term relief.[34]

A Japanese study of aquatic exercise for patients with low-back pain found that 90% of the patients reported improvement after six months. Exercises focused on strengthening the abdominal, gluteal, and leg muscles, stretching back, hip, hamstring, and calf muscles as well as walking in water and swimming. Patients participated from one to three times per week. Those who exercised more often showed a more significant physical improvement than those who exercised less.[35] Another study showed an increased return-to-work rate for people with low-back pain after an aquatic exercise program.[36]

My Exercise Program

I began swimming as part of my back pain recovery program after taking a class at the YMCA to improve my swimming skills. I have been swimming laps at least five times a week for 35 years now. I find it enjoyable and relaxing—a way to keep both mentally and physically healthy. I combine the swimming with daily stretching and limbering exercises and supplement with walking, bicycling, and cross country skiing whenever feasible.

Yoga

Yoga originated in India and is thousands of years old. It was introduced in the United States in 1893.[37] There are many types of yogic practices, some of which focus more on philosophy and others that focus more on physical and mental practice. In the United States the most popular type of yoga is hatha yoga, which includes physical exercises and postures, breathing techniques and meditation.[38] A well designed hatha yoga program increases body awareness, increases muscle strength and flexibility and promotes relaxation.[39]

A systematic review in 2011 of 10 randomized clinical trials of yoga in the treatment of chronic pain found that yoga leads to significantly greater pain reduction than standard care, self-care, therapeutic exercises, touch and manipulation, or no treatment.[40]

A 16-week study using iyengar yoga with patients with more than 10 years of chronic low-back pain found at three-month follow-up that patients had, on average, a 64% reduction in pain intensity, a 77% reduction in functional disability, and an 88% reduction in pain medication usage.[41]

A small, randomized controlled three-month study tested the effectiveness and safety of yoga therapy for adults aged

20 to 45 with nonspecific low-back pain or sciatica and disc extrusions or bulges. Patients participated in group classes and home practice of yoga that was modified to ensure safety for disc extrusions. Yoga was found to reduce pain and disability with no adverse effects.[42]

Yoga is no-impact and is meant to be done slowly with body awareness. Injuries can occur when yoga is taught in large classes with poor supervision.[43] Within hatha yoga are many different styles of yoga, some more gentle and some more strenuous than others. For someone in chronic pain, the safest route, if possible, is to start with one-on -one instruction with a yoga teacher trained in therapeutic yoga techniques. Some forms of yoga that have been specifically developed for therapeutic use include Integrative, Phoenix Rising, and Svaroopa yoga.[44]

Make sure, if you do take a yoga class, that your instructor is paying attention to your efforts and advising appropriate precautions for your condition. When I was in the early stages of my own back pain problem, I injured myself and made my back pain worse in an overcrowded yoga class with an inattentive teacher. She failed to emphasize to us that the safe practice of yoga involves paying attention to limitations and learning to gently expand our capacity.

CHAPTER 10

HOMEOPATHY

Homeopathy is based on the principle that "like cures like." This means that any substance capable of producing symptoms in a healthy person can cure similar symptoms in a person who is sick. This idea is referred to as the "law of similar." For instance, an onion makes your eyes water and your nose burn. If you are having an attack of hay fever with watering eyes and a burning nose, a homeopathic remedy made from onion can relieve it.

A second homeopathy principle is that you should administer the least amount of medicine necessary to evoke a healing response. This is called the "minimum dose." To prevent side effects, Hahnemann began successive dilution with shaking his medicines to find the point at which they would be therapeutic but not toxic. He also discovered that in many situations the best cure was achieved by the highest possible dilution. Homeopathic remedies can be taken orally or used in topical ointments.

Homeopathy has been controversial partly because homeopathic medicines in high potencies are so diluted that theoretically there should be no measurable remnants of the starting materials left. In a 2010 study, researchers demonstrated for the first time the presence of nanoparticles of the original substance in these extreme homeopathic dilutions.[1]

Currently, 3,000 substances are used as homeopathic remedies to treat everything from colds and cough to arthritis and cancer. Homeopaths typically conduct lengthy patient interviews, often lasting one to two hours initially. The homeopath will ask seemingly unrelated questions about everything from how the patient's senses of taste and smell respond to certain foods to how she sleeps. The patient may be asked about memory, sense of humor, and bodily functions, in addition to many very specific questions about lifestyle, behaviors, and health. The answers help the homeopath pinpoint the remedy most likely to be effective.

A Brief History

Homeopathy was developed in 1827 by Dr. Samuel Hahnemann, a German physician. Hahnemann was appalled by the painful and extreme treatments that patients were enduring to combat illness. Common medical treatments of the time included bloodletting, administration of large quantities of laxatives, and administration of emetics, which cause vomiting and heavy sweating. Physicians at that time also used chloroform and large doses of mercury, which is now known to cause brain damage, sometimes in doses of 4 tablespoons or more a day. Another popular treatment was blistering.[2]

Natalie Robins describes the history of homeopathy in her book *Copeland's Cure*. Because of its painlessness, lack of side effects, and relative simplicity, homeopathy "caught on like wildfire across America."[3] Heightened interest in homeopathy began during the cholera epidemics of 1832 and 1849 when many people noticed that this new treatment option was more effective and more pleasant than the conventional treatment with chloroform. Patients appreciated that homeopathic doctors spent more time listening to them and that their remedies were gentle and effective.

As the interest in homeopathy grew, the first homeopathic medical schools were established. There were 44 in the United States by the end of the 19th century. It wasn't long before some of these medical schools, unhappy with the state of existing hospitals, opened hospitals of their own. There were more than 100 homeopath-supervised hospitals by 1892.

The deadly swine flu pandemic of 1918–1919 showed how powerful homeopathic remedies and principles could be. During an epidemic that killed 22 million people worldwide, deaths in patients treated with homeopathy were rare.[4]

Epidemiological and anecdotal evidence of the effectiveness of homeopathy did not deter efforts by the conventional medical community to eliminate the practice of it. In fact, the war waged by conventional practitioners against homeopaths began soon after the birth of homeopathic medicine.

Homeopaths created the first medical association in the United States, the American Institute of Homeopathy, in 1844. Its first members were graduates of the same leading medical schools as their counterpart conventional practitioners. It was only later that they became converts to homeopathy. Still, when the American Medical Association (AMA) was formed just three years later, one of its first actions was to ban homeopaths from becoming members. The AMA also decreed that its members would risk expulsion if they consulted with a homeopath. One doctor who consulted with his wife who was studying to become a homeopath was expelled from his local medical society.[5] This was the beginning of the PR and legal and political campaign of war against homeopaths that eventually succeeded in closing every homeopathic medical school and hospital in the United States.

Homeopathy Today

Despite more than a century of aggressive, targeted efforts to discredit and ultimately eliminate homeopathy, it is experiencing a resurgence in the United States today. This interest has been fueled by consumer interest in safer medical treatments. In much of Europe—particularly Great Britain, France, and Germany—homeopathy has, since its inception, been a well-accepted, popular option for the treatment and prevention of a broad range of health conditions.

Traumeel, a topical ointment that contains 12 homeopathic remedies, has been available over the counter in Germany for over 60 years and is currently available in more than 50 countries. Traumeel was demonstrated in a 1989 doubled-blind randomized controlled study to speed healing of acute ankle sprains, including restoration of full range of motion and resolution of pain during movement.[6] Traumeel is frequently used with good to very good results in acute musculoskeletal injuries as well as for degenerative and inflammatory conditions such as osteoarthritis, frozen shoulder, carpal tunnel syndrome, and tennis elbow, according to multicenter drug surveillance studies in Europe. It works as well, or better, than NSAIDs, with no adverse effects.[7]

In the United States, homeopathic remedies are regulated by the FDA. Thanks to the efforts of homeopathic physician Royal Copeland, the US Senator from New York when the Federal Food, Drug, and Cosmetic Act was passed in 1936, homeopathy's own standards, as expressed in the *Homoeopathic Pharmacopoeia of the United States* (HPUS), were incorporated as part of the act.[8] Homeopathic remedies are generally recognized as safe. Most are sold over the counter. They can be found in health food stores and online.

There are currently relatively few homeopathic practitioners in the United States. Since homeopathic remedies are not toxic, it's safe to try them on your own if you can't find a practitioner. There are many books, and even apps, that can help you pinpoint the appropriate remedy, such as *Homeopathy for Musculoskeletal Healing* by Dr. Asa Hershoff.[9]

In recent years, there has been an orchestrated attempt to discredit and ban homeopathy in Europe. In the United Kingdom, four homeopathic hospitals are currently part of the National Health Service (NHS), the government-run system of care. Several others have closed in recent years. Patients can ask their doctor to refer them to one of these hospitals, but it is up to the doctor to decide whether or not to grant these requests. Many doctors have stopped referring patients to homeopathic hospitals.

Agencies called Primary Care Trusts (PCTs) work with local authorities and other agencies to provide free health and social care on a local level. The country has 151 PCTs, and they control 80 percent of the NHS budget. All patient referrals must be approved by the patient's PCT.

Figures obtained in 2007 by *The Times* (London) under the Freedom of Information Act showed that 86 PCTs had either stopped or seriously restricted referrals to Britain's homeopathic hospitals.[10] The number of PCTs restricting access to homeopathic hospitals has continued to grow, and there are several factors that have contributed to this.

In August of 2005, the very prestigious medical journal *The Lancet* featured an anonymous editorial entitled "The End of Homeopathy." Doctors were encouraged to be "bold and honest with their patients about homoeopathy's lack of benefit".[11] The issue also included a meta-analysis (referred to as the Shang study) that stated that homeopathy was no better than a placebo. The study concluded that "biases are present in placebo-controlled trials of both homoeopathy and conventional medicine. When account was taken for these biases in the analysis, there was weak evidence for a specific effect of homoeopathic remedies, but strong evidence for specific effects of conventional interventions. This finding is compatible with the notion that the clinical effects of homoeopathy are placebo effects."[12]

According to homeopath Carol Boyce, "Since that well-planned 'End of Homeopathy' issue of *The Lancet*, there has been a relentless attack on homeopathy in the UK media. . . . The impact has been huge; the fallout extensive. After all, *The Lancet* is one of the oldest peer-reviewed medical journals in the world. This issue of *The Lancet* was a coup of the highest order. The Shang et al. meta-analysis can be dismantled by anyone willing to read the entire paper and not simply the title and conclusion. Of the 110 trials of homoeopathy that matched the study's criteria, the authors reached their conclusion by using just eight trials—and the eight used were not identified in the published paper! At the insistence of members of the homoeopathic medical community, the eight trials were eventually revealed, and it became clear that extreme "cherry-picking" had transpired; only these eight particular trials would lead to a negative result. A meta-analysis using other combinations of the 110 trials available would weigh in favour of homoeopathy."[13]

About six months after the Lancet articles were released, 13 of the UK's most prominent medical professionals sent letters to PCTs urging them to stop referring patients for CAM treatments such as homeopathy. The letter began with an introduction that said, "We are a group of physicians and scientists who are concerned about ways in which unproven or disproved treatments are being encouraged for general use in the NHS. There is now overt promotion of homeopathy in parts of the NHS. It is an implausible treatment for which over a dozen systematic reviews have failed to produce convincing evidence of effectiveness."[14] The letter was leaked to the media and appeared on the front page of *The Times*.

The most prominent homeopathic hospital in England is the Royal London Homeopathic Hospital (RLHH). According to Dr. Ian Fisher, personal homeopath to the Queen and clinical director of the RLHH, the hospital was affected by what he calls "an orchestrated campaign" against alternative medicine by some of Britain's most distinguished doctors".[15] In 2007, he wrote an open letter to his fellow countrymen asking for help in saving the RLHH from closure. He said that the hospital, founded in 1849, was in danger of closing because PCTs had stopped or drastically reduced their funding of treatment at the RLHH. In an interview, Fisher said that he believed that this was happening because PCTs felt pressured after receiving the letter that was written by the 13 prominent British doctors in 2006.[16]

A once bustling hospital that included inpatient and surgical wards, the RLHH is now home to only about 20 doctors. Despite their critics, these doctors continue to believe in what they are doing. According to Dr. Sarah Eames, director of women's services at the hospital, "I have been a doctor for over 30 years. I worked as a GP before I stumbled across homeopathy like most people here. What we specialize in is people who are not helped by conventional medicine. Their suffering is long term and we can save money on NHS tests and treatment that has not proved particularly helpful."[17] With regard to the skepticism surrounding homeopathy, she says, "It may be dismissed as anecdote but when you continue to see people respond it does build up. Homeopathy has been going for 200 years and hundreds of thousands of people have been treated. Do you discount them all?"[18]

In response to the mounting negative publicity surrounding homeopathy—one prominent doctor referred to it as "witchcraft" in 2010—the RLHH made the decision to change their name. The institution that operated under the same name for over 100 years is now called the Royal London Hospital for Integrated Medicine.

Similar efforts are underway in Germany, the country where homeopathy originated.

Homeopathy does not lend itself to the types of research studies used for prescription drugs—in which everyone with the same symptom gets the same drug—because homeopathic treatment is, by definition, individualized. This is based on the principle that the total person, rather than a specific symptom, must be treated. This makes traditional clinical trials very difficult and makes it easy to design a study that seems to show that homeopathy is ineffective. Another obstacle is the lack of funding sources for studies of homeopathy and other forms of alternative medicine.

Research Results

Despite these barriers, numerous studies have shown the effectiveness of homeopathy in treating chronic pain, including pain from rheumatoid arthritis, osteoarthritis, fibromyalgia, and muscle pain. Many of these studies have met the gold standard of research: they are randomized controlled double-blind studies.

In a 1980 randomized controlled double-blind study of homeopathy in the treatment of rheumatoid arthritis, patients with rheumatoid arthritis were given either an individualized homeopathic remedy or a placebo in addition to their standard care with anti-inflammatory drugs. The homeopathic treatment group showed significant improvements in joint tenderness, limbering up time, grip strength, and pain compared to the group receiving the placebo. There were no adverse effects of the homeopathic remedies.[19]

A 1987 Italian study of homeopathic treatment of migraine headaches—also a double-blinded randomized controlled study—found that individualized homeopathic treatment significantly reduced severity, frequency, and duration of migraine headaches compared to a placebo. The average severity in the treatment group after a period of four months of homeopathic dosing at four separate times over four week intervals was reduced from 9.1 to 2.9 on a 10 point scale in the homeopathic treatment group compared to a reduction from 8.4 to 7.8 in the placebo group. Migraine frequency was reduced from a mean of 10 times per month to 1.8 in the treatment group compared to a reduction from 9.9 to 7.9 in the placebo group. Duration of migraine attacks decreased in the treatment group from 19.9 hours to 6.7 hours compared to a reduction from 18.6 hours to 17.9 hours in the placebo group.[20]

A homeopathic treatment group was compared with a group of patients taking Acetaminophen in a randomized controlled double-blinded study of osteoarthritis in 1998. The homeopathic treatment was found to produce significantly better pain relief than the Acetaminophen, with no adverse effects.[21]

A 2004 randomized double blinded, controlled study found that homeopathic treatment was significantly better than a placebo in reducing tender point pain, improving quality of life and overall health and reducing depression in patients with fibromyalgia.[22]

The homeopathic drug combination called Lymphdiaral basistophen was studied in a 2012 German double-blind, randomized placebo-controlled study. The homeopathic treatment significantly improved functional ability of patients with low-back pain compared to a placebo. The patients took the remedy three times daily over a 105-day period. All patients in the study also received inpatient naturopathic treatment. The incidence of adverse reactions was similar in both the treatment and placebo groups.[23]

A 2014 comprehensive review and meta-analysis of all available literature on the homeopathic treatment of fibromyalgia, which included case reports as well as randomized controlled trials, found an overall positive effect. The authors believed the evidence was strong enough for homeopathy to be considered a complementary treatment for fibromyalgia, though they stated that the findings were still preliminary.[24]

CHAPTER 11

ACUPUNCTURE

Acupuncture is a treatment system that involves inserting thin needles into specific points on the body in order to positively affect a patient's health. Acupuncture is a therapy that has been developed and refined over thousands of years and is part of traditional Chinese medicine (TCM). Treatment is focused on the individual, not the diagnosis, and the goal is to treat the root cause of the problem and the reasons why the individual cannot heal.[1]

TCM is based on the principle that the universe is balanced between two opposing forces, yin and yang. Yin is soft, dark, cold, lower, passive, nourishing, and still. Yang, its opposite, is hard, bright, hot, upper, dominant, consuming, and active. The interaction of these two forces is believed to create qi (pronounced "chee"), the vital energy that is life itself. Qi flows through the body along energy pathways known as meridians. The meridians are believed to be related to different organs. Along each meridian are many points that are stimulated through the insertion and manipulation of the acupuncture needles to regulate the flow of qi. There are 361 acupuncture points in classic Chinese medicine. Over time, many different styles of acupuncture have been developed, with more than 2,000 acupoints currently identified.[2]

Traditionally, needles are manipulated by pecking, twirling, and flicking until the patient feels sensations of soreness, heaviness and/or tingling. More recently developed applications of acupuncture include electroacupuncture (stimulating the inserted needles with small electric currents) and laser acupuncture (stimulating the acupoints with light). Points are also traditionally stimulated with moxibustion (burning a small amount of an herb) and cupping (using a special glass cup to create a vacuum in order to move stagnant blood and qi).[3]

Many Americans first heard about acupuncture in 1971 when Henry Kissinger, President Nixon's secretary of state, visited China after the resumption of diplomatic relations between the two countries. James Reston, a journalist working for the *New York Times* who accompanied Kissinger, experienced acute appendicitis while in China, necessitating emergency surgery. During his recovery, he was treated with acupuncture for pain and wrote about his experience for the newspaper.[4]

Acupuncture in the United States

Even before Reston raised awareness about acupuncture in the United States, Chinese immigrants trained in acupuncture were quietly practicing it, even though the practice was illegal here. Miriam Lee, who trained as a nurse–midwife and acupuncturist before coming to the United States in 1966, worked on an assembly line in California while giving acupuncture treatments out of her home and later at a supportive doctor's office. In 1974, Lee joined the unfortunately large ranks of immigrants arrested for practicing medicine without a license. Her patients packed the courtroom at her trial and demanded their right to the only medical treatment that had helped them. A few days later, then-California Governor Ronald Reagan legally authorized acupuncture as an experimental procedure that could be practiced under the supervision of a licensed physician for research purposes. One year later, California became the first state in the United States to legalize acupuncture.[5] Today, 46 states regulate the legal practice of acupuncture. The exceptions are Alabama, Kansas, North Dakota, South Dakota, Oklahoma, and Wyoming.[6]

In 2007, it was estimated that 3 million American adults used acupuncture each year.[7] The most common reason for visiting an acupuncturist was for treatment of chronic pain.[8] Most patients self-refer for acupuncture instead of receiving physician referrals.[9]

Most acupuncturists in the United States are not physicians but have three or four years of acupuncture training, which results in a master's degree.[10] Most states also require that nonphysician acupuncturists pass a national exam administered by the National Commission for the Certification of Acupuncture and Oriental Medicine.[11] Training courses for physicians wishing to practice acupuncture are available and consist of 200 to 300 hours of training. Most acupuncturists also engage in postgraduate training.[12]

Research Results

Acupuncture has been the subject of significant research, including research into its underlying mechanisms and its effect on clinical conditions, including pain. Studies have shown that acupuncture affects the supply of neurochemicals, including levels of endorphins, cortisol, serotonin, and dopamine.[13] Other studies have shown changes in levels of brain activity with needling of acupuncture points.[14]

There is currently not enough data to determine the number of needles, length of treatment session, frequency of treatment, or total number of sessions required for effective treatment. Depending on the condition, experienced acupuncturists recommend 1 to 3 treatments a week of 20-to-30-minute sessions, using a minimum of 6 to 11 needles each time for 6 to 10 treatments for a positive result. Studies of acupuncture have used anywhere from 2 to 20 needles per session of 4 to 30 minutes, with frequency ranging from biweekly to three times per week and total number of treatments ranging from 1 to 40 sessions.[15]

As with other forms of alternative medicine, such as nutrition and biofeedback, studies that include inadequate doses of a treatment (treatment sessions too few in number or too short, or insufficient amount of a substance) or inadequately trained providers seem designed to discredit the treatment rather than to shed light on whether it actually works. Fortunately, there has been an increase in recent years of well-designed studies of acupuncture treatment. These studies show that acupuncture is an effective treatment for chronic pain and many other conditions.

One review of available evidence of the effectiveness of acupuncture for chronic pain looked at eight meta-analyses that were published between 2003 and 2008. The researchers concluded that there is consistent evidence that acupuncture for knee osteoarthritis and headache is more effective than placebo (sham acupuncture) for both short-term and long-term pain relief. For chronic back pain, they found that acupuncture is more effective than placebo for short-term relief. But studies were inconsistent regarding long-term effectiveness.[16]

In a 2012 study that included individual patient data from 29 controlled studies with a total of 17,922 patients, researchers concluded that acupuncture is an effective treatment for chronic back and neck pain, osteoarthritis, and chronic headaches.[17]

A 2007 German study of 1,162 patients compared acupuncture, sham acupuncture (superficial needling at nonacupuncture points), and conventional therapy (a combination of drugs, physical therapy, and exercise) for effectiveness against low-back pain. The study concluded that both acupuncture and sham acupuncture were almost twice as effective as conventional treatment for chronic back pain. The improvements lasted at least six months.[18]

Acupuncture modestly improved pain and stiffness in fibromyalgia sufferers in a 2013 Cochrane review. Sham acupuncture seemed to reduce pain and fatigue and improve sleep and overall well-being as well as real acupuncture. The review also found that electroacupuncture was better than the manual variety for reducing pain, stiffness, and fatigue and for improving sleep and global well-being in fibromyalgia sufferers. Acupuncture also seemed to enhance the effects of medication and exercise in reducing fibromyalgia symptoms. Improvements lasted at least 1 month but were not generally still present at 6 months. The review also concluded that acupuncture appeared to be a safe treatment for fibromyalgia.[19]

The World Health Organization states that acupuncture is safe if it is properly performed by a well-trained practitioner. WHO reported that acupuncture is nontoxic and that adverse reactions are minimal. Effects on pain were found to be comparable to morphine without the side effects and risks.[20]

A Practitioner's Experience

Philomena Kong, MD, who now practices acupuncture in upstate New York, grew up in Hong Kong, where her great-grandfather, grandfather, and mother practiced traditional Chinese medicine, including acupuncture. She often assisted them in their work. During what she describes as a period of "rebelliousness," and with a desire to practice "scientific medicine," she came to the United States and attended pharmacy school. After practicing as a pharmacist for a couple of years, she went to medical school in Texas and then specialized in physical and rehabilitation medicine. Kong worked at a hospital in upstate New York for a few years but was dissatisfied because she had very little patient contact after the initial assessment of a patient. She decided to get trained and licensed as an acupuncturist in New York State. Her training involved coursework in the United States as well as internships in China and France. She has now been practicing exclusively as an acupuncturist for more than 20 years.

Most of Kong's patients seek out her acupuncture services for chronic pain. Because of her background, Kong often works closely with physical therapists and reported that the two treatments complement each other well. She reported that acupuncture can often increase range of motion, which increases the effectiveness of physical therapy intervention. She has also found that acupuncture is a good complement to other alternative modalities, such as chiropractic and massage. Unfortunately, financial limitations and lack of insurance coverage often keep patients from pursuing multiple treatment modalities.

Kong also reported that in her experience, acupuncture is a good standalone treatment, even for such treatment-resistant problems as chronic low-back pain. Different patients respond differently to treatment, with some responding more quickly than others. She has found that most back pain patients respond well within four to six sessions.

Lee

Dr. Kong cited one dramatic example of a patient I'll call Lee who came in on crutches. His doctor had recommended back surgery, but he was resistant. At the end of his first acupuncture session, Lee was able to walk out of her office without the crutches. He did not have the back surgery and only came back again much later to see her when he had a new problem to be treated.

Kong also reported that many of her patients can decrease their use of pain medications, including opioids. In fact, many come to see her specifically for that purpose.

Some insurance plans have become more restrictive in their coverage of acupuncture in recent years, according to Kong, especially New York State workers' compensation plans. Other insurances have started to cover acupuncture, but most still don't.[21]

CHAPTER 12
ENERGY HEALING

Western medicine focuses on the concrete level of the physical body. The interventions used—pharmaceuticals, surgery, radiation, gene therapy—all zero in on changing structure and function at this level. Mind/body interventions, such as meditation, biofeedback, and psychotherapy, target a second dimension of human experience: thoughts, feelings, and beliefs. Treatments focusing on the mind/body connection are gradually gaining more acceptance in mainstream medicine. There is yet a third dimension of human experience widely acknowledged by traditional healing systems, such as Chinese medicine and ayurvedic (Indian) medicine, known as vital energy, spirit, or subtle energy. Because there is no theoretical framework in Western medicine for this concept, alternative medicine approaches that are energy based are the most controversial.[1]

Some of the interventions covered in previous chapters—including acupuncture, homeopathy, and energy psychology techniques—work on the energy level to promote healing. There is another group of interventions that use "laying on of the hands" to facilitate healing, including of chronic pain. The most well-known are therapeutic touch and Reiki.

Therapeutic touch (TT) was developed in the early 1970s by registered nurse Dolores Krieger. The basis of TT is that there is an energy field within the human body that can cause illnesses and other physical problems if it becomes imbalanced. TT practitioners are trained to use their hands to detect the body's energy fields and to correct, or balance, these fields. Advocates believe that it can promote self-healing, reduce pain, and promote relaxation. Krieger has personally trained tens of thousands of practitioners, primarily nurses, and her trainees have since trained many others. Krieger is currently a professor emerita in nursing science at New York University.[2]

As with the other so-called alternative treatments for pain, there has been a backlash from the mainstream medical community. The bias against energy healing is shown by the very different treatment of two researchers who reached opposite conclusions about energy healing.

The Case of Dr. Gloria Gronowicz

Dr. Gloria Gronowicz, a researcher and professor in the department of surgery at the University of Connecticut, never expected to get involved in the TT debate. After receiving her doctorate in cell biology from Columbia University, she has spent more than 20 years studying the biology of bone cells. She is a respected researcher who has published more than 80 papers in her field.

Several years ago, Gronowicz was approached by a colleague and asked to conduct a study on the effect of TT on bone cells. Although she had no previous interest or experience with TT, she says, "I characterize myself as open-minded, and I love new ideas. I always hear people out, and I had a lot of respect for her [the colleague]." Despite the fact that she was very willing to participate in the study, she was quick to admit that she did not expect TT to have any effect in a laboratory setting. She described all of her work up until that time as "mainstream."

Gronowicz applied to the NIH for a grant to fund an experiment designed to determine if TT could have any effect on bone cell cultures. After being turned down once, she ended up receiving a grant from the NIH for $250,000.

With funding in place, she began her study. She placed three groups of bone cell cultures in petri dishes and kept them in incubators. Twice a week for three years trained TT practitioners arrived at the lab and removed one dish of cells from the incubator and held their hands above it for 10 minutes. (TT practitioners do not actually touch their patients; they hold their hands several inches from their bodies.) The practitioners themselves admitted that it was very strange for them to work this way, but they did their best to treat the petri dish as if it were an actual patient.

Students with no background in TT arrived at the lab at the same frequency and held their hands over a second dish of cell cultures. A third dish of cultures was simply ignored. The studies were conducted on healthy bone cells and bone-cancer cells.

The scientists who analyzed the cells under a microscope had no idea which group of cells received which sort of treatment. Much to the shock of Gronowicz, they discovered that the healthy cells treated by trained TT practitioners grew faster and stronger than those in the other two groups. "Therapeutic touch stimulated growth in bone, tendon, and skin cells at statistically significant rates," said Gronowicz. She also noted that the cells absorbed more calcium, a necessary mineral for maintaining strong bones.

To confirm her results, she tested the cells using several different biological markers for growth. Each test confirmed her original laboratory findings. "I was so astounded by the results," said Gronowicz. "I wasn't expecting any results. I was very shocked."

Meanwhile, when the bone-cancer cells were studied, it was discovered that TT had no effect on their growth. This was also considered good news for the field of TT because stimulating the growth of cancer cells would harm patients.

Once Gronowicz's study was complete, she began submitting her final research paper to medical journals for publication. With her scientific background, credibility, and publication experience, getting one of her studies published in a respected journal had never been a problem for her. She discovered that was not the case when it came to a study on such a controversial area of complementary and alternative medicine.

Her work was rejected without adequate explanation by several journals. After she submitted her work to the *Journal of Orthopaedic Research*, the editors sent her a long list of questions related to the study. After she provided them with six or seven pages of detailed responses to their questions, she received a letter saying that her paper had been rejected.

It wasn't until she called the editor and persuaded him to reconsider his decision that her work was finally published in 2008.[3] At his request, she agreed to rerun some of her statistical calculations before publication. She freely admits that her work would have never been published if not for the scientific credibility that she had established during her more than 20 years as a researcher.

After her study was published, she went to a meeting also attended by the editor of the *Journal of Orthopaedic Research*. She thanked him for "going out on a limb" and publishing her work when no one else would. He told her that he received a great deal of criticism from his colleagues and readers for making that decision.

Regarding the negative reaction among her own colleagues, she says, "I think that we are not as unbiased as we say that we are as scientists."

She says that the day that her study was featured on the front page of the *Hartford Courant* (July 28, 2008), "The people that I worked with in the bone group [at the university] for twenty years did not say a word about it. It was shocking to me that no one acknowledged it. It is very hard for me to understand. I think that this [her TT research] is fundamentally against some people's views. It is like saying that the world is flat."

At one point, one of her colleagues told her that she should be more careful when choosing her research projects. "I was told that people would think that I was crazy," Gronowicz says.

Today, she would like to work on more research projects related to TT and is "trying desperately to get funded." She continues to experience what she describes as "such prejudice" when applying for grants for TT studies. According to her, this prejudice exists even within the CAM field where TT is controversial.

She has no regrets about getting involved with TT. "I am a tenured professor, and we should be doing risky science," she said. "I have always been more open-minded than a lot of other people, so I feel that I was the right person to do this."[4]

The Case of Emily Rosa

Ten years before Gronowicz struggled to get study results published, a different type of TT study made headlines. This study was not done by a well-respected scientist—it was done by a fourth grader as a science project. At the age of nine, Emily Rosa conducted a study to see if therapeutic touch practitioners could detect a human energy field. She recruited 21 practitioners and asked them to sit behind a screen so that they could not see her. She then asked them to stick their hands through an opening in the screen. She held one of her hands over one of their hands—she determined which hand by flipping a coin—and they were to tell her which one of their hands detected Emily's energy force. The results of the study showed that the practitioners were correct only 44% of the time.

With help from her mother, Rosa wrote a report on her study. According to an article in *TIME* magazine, "Her mother Linda Rosa, a registered nurse, has been campaigning against TT for nearly a decade, and her stepfather Larry Sarner is chairman of the National Therapeutic Touch Study Group, an anti-TT organization."[5]

Rosa's study concluded: "Twenty-one experienced TT practitioners were unable to detect the investigator's energy field. Their failure to substantiate TT's most fundamental claim is unrefuted evidence that the claims of TT are groundless and that further professional use is unjustified."

Her study was published in 1998 in the *Journal of the American Medical Association (JAMA),*[6] and she was featured on ABC News, Fox News, and NPR. Many newspapers also reported on her study, including the *New York Times.*[7]

The Rosa study was much criticized by *JAMA* readers because they thought the research methods were inappropriate.[8] In addition, all of the study authors were strongly biased against therapeutic touch, including coauthor Stephen Barrett, MD. A retired psychiatrist, Barrett runs several websites criticizing alternative medicine, the best known of which is Quackwatch.com. Barrett defines *quackery* as "anything involving overpromotion in the field of health," but he does not criticize conventional medicine because it's "way outside his scope."[9]

Several years after the publication of Rosa's study, an article criticizing the statistical analysis in the study was published by a nurse–statistician. Besides pointing out statistical fallacies in the original analysis, she noted that none of the authors had any credentials in statistical analysis.[10] Of course, the general public did not see any of the criticisms of the study and was left with the impression that therapeutic touch is a fraud.

Other Research Results

Just a year after Rosa's study was published, a 1999 meta-analysis of 13 controlled studies of therapeutic touch for various conditions showed moderate positive effects.[11]

A 2008 Cochrane review of touch therapies for pain relief in adults included 24 randomized controlled trials and controlled clinical trials that included 1,153 participants. The review evaluated the effects of touch therapies on any type of pain. Modalities included were healing touch, therapeutic touch, and Reiki. They found on average a modest reduction of pain. More experienced practitioners and Reiki practitioners achieved the best results.[12]

A 2014 study reviewed randomized controlled trials of nontouch biofield therapies—therapeutic touch, healing touch, external qigong, and Reiki—in which the practitioner works with the patient's energy field without actually touching the patient. Many of the studies reviewed included only one treatment session, for as little as five minutes The authors concluded that there were enough significant positive findings from the available research to justify funding of larger studies that could yield more definitive data.[13]

According to a 2005 survey by the American Hospital Association, 30% of hospitals were offering therapeutic touch to patients at that time.[14] Despite that fact that mainstream medicine practitioners still consider energy healing approaches unproven, patients want these types of treatments and they believe they benefit from them.

CHAPTER 13
MARIJUANA

Marijuana grows wild in all but the coldest climates all around the world. The first known written reference to the use of marijuana, also known as cannabis and hemp, for medical use was by Chinese Emperor Shen Nung in 2737 BCE. He recommended marijuana for treatment of gout, rheumatism, female weakness, malaria, constipation, beriberi, and absent-mindedness.[1]

Medical Research Versus Policy

The United States Pharmacopeia (USP), created in 1820, is a nonprofit organization that sets federal standards of quality for medicines, dietary supplements, and foods. From its inception until 1941, cannabis was listed in the US Pharmacopoeia as an appropriate medication for treating migraine headaches, fatigue, rheumatism, asthma, coughing fits, delirium tremens, and menstrual symptoms. Many pharmaceutical companies—including Squibb, Parke-Davis, and Lilly—produced tinctures and elixirs containing cannabis that were consumed by Americans of all ages.[2] During this time, cannabis was widely available without a prescription.[3] In 1941, cannabis was removed from the USP at the request of Federal Bureau of Narcotics Commissioner Harry Anslinger, a virulent antimarijuana crusader.[4]

The LaGuardia Report, commissioned by New York City's then-mayor and published in 1944, found that marijuana use did not lead to addiction, dependence upon opiates, juvenile delinquency, or serious criminal behavior, and that it might have therapeutic applications.[5] The AMA, previously a strong supporter of the medical uses of marijuana, after intense lobbying by Commissioner Anslinger, did an abrupt about-face and came out against the LaGuardia Report, calling it "unscientific."[6,7] In 2009, the AMA again reversed its stance, urging that marijuana be removed from the Schedule 1 (most restricted) category of drugs, in the hope that this would facilitate research on medical marijuana.[8]

A 1999 federal Institute of Medicine review that found that marijuana was helpful in reducing chemotherapy-induced nausea and AIDS wasting, among other conditions. Despite this, in 2006, the FDA declared, "There are no sound scientific studies" supporting the medical use of marijuana.[9]

Dr. Jerry Avon, professor of medicine at Harvard Medical School, said of the FDA's pronouncement, "Unfortunately, this is yet another example of the FDA making pronouncements that seem to be driven more by ideology than by science."[10]

The FDA also held that state legislation to legalize medical marijuana was not consistent with the FDA's requirements that medications undergo the rigorous FDA approval process. Many experts interviewed by the *New York Times* on this subject reported that it was near impossible to get high-quality marijuana for research purposes or funding for studies of marijuana from the federal government, making the conduct of studies to prove benefits extremely difficult.[11]

The US government has refused to make research-grade marijuana available for privately funded research and has prohibited private laboratories from producing it for scientific research even in the face of advisory court opinions that it do so. Other similarly classified controlled substances—such as heroin, cocaine, LSD, and MMDA (ecstasy)—are all available to researchers from DEA-licensed laboratories.[12]

The FDA has, however, approved dronabinol (brand name Marinol), a synthetic form of one of marijuana's components, delta-9-tetrahydrocannabinol (THC), to treat nausea in cancer chemotherapy patients in 1985. In 1992, the FDA also approved Marinol to stimulate appetite in AIDS patients with wasting syndrome.[13] But dronabinol has the following side effects:[14]

- Dizziness
- Nausea
- Drowsiness
- Inability to focus
- Unsteady gait
- Mood changes
- Confusion
- Delusions
- Hallucinations

Psychoactive effects of dronabinol ingestion after two hours were found to be similar to the psychoactive effects of smoking marijuana after 30 minutes.[15]

Another synthetic form of THC, cesamet (brand name Nabilone) was approved by the FDA for nausea and vomiting caused by chemotherapy. Cesamet was originally approved by the FDA for use in the United States in 1985, but it was removed from the market until reapproved by the FDA in 2006. Cesamet was also approved in the United Kingdom and Australia (1982), Canada (1981), and Mexico (2007).[16]

Another pharmaceutical, Sativex, was approved in the United Kingdom in 2010 to treat neuropathic pain and spasticity in multiple sclerosis patients and moderate to severe pain in advanced cancer patients. Sativex is made from two natural extracts of the marijuana plant, THC and cannabidiol (CBD). It was subsequently approved and is currently in Phase III trials in the United States for treatment of cancer pain:[17] Sativex has already been approved in the following countries:

- Spain
- Canada
- Czech Republic
- Denmark
- Germany
- Sweden
- Austria
- Italy
- Switzerland
- Finland
- Israel
- Norway
- Poland

Cannabinoids Are Found Only in Marijuana and Mammals

The marijuana plant contains more than 100 substances known as cannabinoids, which are unique to the plant. The most well-known are THC and CBD.[18] The brains of mammals also produce substances known as endocannabinoids, which have been referred to as "the brain's own marijuana."[19] Whether they are produced by the body (endogenous) or derived from plants or synthetic formulations (exogenous), cannabinoids bind with receptors on cells throughout the body to create their effects.[20] These cannabinoid receptors are involved in metabolic regulation, craving, pain, anxiety, bone growth, and immune function.[21] The cannabinoid's interaction with cannabinoid receptors in the brain stem and spinal cord is responsible for their effect on pain.[22]

The body releases endocannabinoids in response to muscle spasm, spasticity, inflammation,[23] and traumatic stress.[24]

Whole plant marijuana is considered superior by many to its synthesized components, such as THC in Marinol. Marijuana has a broad spectrum of therapeutic effects because of its many different cannabinoids.[25] The elevated mood achieved by smoking marijuana in addition to relief from symptoms combines to create a feeling of improved well-being.[26] Synthesized THC that is ingested, as in Marinol, can take an hour or more to take effect. The psychological effects, which are more intense and more unpredictable, can last up to three times longer than when exposure to THC is achieved through smoking marijuana.[27]

Research Results

A 2011 review of randomized controlled studies of cannabinoids—including whole marijuana, marijuana extract, and synthetic cannabinoids for treatment of chronic, noncancer pain—found significant modest effects on pain relief as well as significant improvements in sleep. No serious adverse effects were reported. Most of the studies reviewed were of neuropathic pain, but one study each of fibromyalgia and rheumatoid arthritis also reported positive results.[28]

A 2015 review of controlled studies of cannabinoids in the treatment of chronic neuropathic pain included studies of marijuana, marijuana extracts, and synthetic cannabinoids. The authors concluded that cannabinoids provide significant pain relief in chronic neuropathic pain in conditions where other treatments do not work. They found that reported side effects in the reviewed studies were minor.[29]

A survey of 100 consecutive medical marijuana patients who were returning for their annual recertification in Hawaii found that 97% used marijuana primarily for relief of chronic pain. They reported an average 64% decrease in pain—a decrease on a 10-point pain scale from 7.8 to 2.8. Half also reported relief from stress and anxiety; 45% reported insomnia relief; and 71% reported no negative side effects. No serious adverse effects were reported. Some of the patients reported they were able to reduce or eliminate their use of opioids.[30]

After research found that CBD reduced the euphoria associated with THC, marijuana growers apparently used genetic engineering to reduce CBD in marijuana and increase concentrations of THC. Researchers examining the components of marijuana seized by law enforcement in California found increases in THC, from 2.17% to 9.93%, while CBD concentrations decreased from 0.24% to 0.08% between 1996 and 2008.[31] CBD appears to alleviate many of THC's negative effects, including acute anxiety that can occur at high doses,[32] and has a better safety profile than THC has.[33]

Smoked marijuana does have safety concerns, especially in those who use heavily and long term, or who started using marijuana early in life. Risks include the following:[34]

- Damage to airways and lungs
- Higher rates of heart attacks
- Increased cardiovascular mortality
- Reduced brain volume
- Reduced fertility
- Depression and suicidal ideation and behavior
- Psychosis
- Impairment of attention, concentration, inhibition, impulsivity, and working memory
- Cognitive impairment of the fetus and reduced fetal growth (pregnant smokers)

There have been rare reports of transient psychotic symptoms or acute psychosis, usually in individuals with a history of mental illness, after smoking marijuana.[35] It is also not advisable for individuals intoxicated by marijuana to operate motor vehicles.[36]

In contrast, CBD is not associated with any toxic side effects, with the exception of sedation and immunosuppression, at higher doses.[37]

Respiratory side effects of smoking marijuana can be significantly reduced by using a vaporizer, according to a 2007 study. Vaporizers heat the marijuana to release the cannabinoids but stay cool enough to eliminate the smoke and toxins that result from burning the marijuana.[38]

Long-term exposure to marijuana smoke has been suspected as a cancer risk, especially for respiratory cancers and mouth, tongue, and esophagus cancers. However, a 2006 study found no connection between these cancers and smoking marijuana, even among heavy smokers. The researcher, Dr. Donald Taskin, theorized that THC has a protective effect against cancer.[39]

In fact, evidence has been accumulating for approximately forty years that marijuana has anticarcinogenic properties, beginning with a study published in 1975 in the *Journal of the National Cancer Institute that* found cannabinoids reduced the progression of lung cancer in rats.[40] The researchers also found that the cannabinoids reduced spleen inflammation associated with leukemia and that when bone marrow was treated with THC, it showed a resistance to cancer that was increased at higher doses.[41] A subsequent study found that THC reduced many types of cancer in mice, including cancers of the breast, uterus, pancreas, and testicles. Higher doses provided greater protection from cancer and led to longer life.[42]

Marijuana may also protect against Alzheimer's disease. In 2006, researchers at the Scripps Institute in California reported that THC is more effective at preventing Alzheimer's disease than any other known substance. The discovery of the way that THC works to prevent the progression of Alzheimer's disease, study author Kim Janda reported, is a "previously unrecognized molecular mechanism" and an important medical breakthrough.[43]

An excellent review of the research on the anticarcinogenic and neuroprotective effects of marijuana can be found in *Marijuana, Gateway to Health: How Cannabis Protects Us from Cancer and Alzheimer's Disease* by Clint Werner.[44] Werner called the aversion to using marijuana as medicine "euphoranoia," an irrational fear of getting high. Werner stated, "There is no justification for keeping the public in the dark about marijuana's medical value when there are so many legal drugs that are much more dangerous to both our physical and mental health."[45]

There is not one single published case of human death worldwide from cannabis poisoning.[46] In fact, research has shown that when used as an adjunct to opiates, cannabinoids provide greater pain relief, which can result in a reduction in opiate use and lower mortality from opiate overdose.[47]

A 2002 study in mice found that coadministering THC with morphine prevented development of morphine tolerance and dependence.[48]

A 2009 study found that medical marijuana users substitute marijuana for more harmful drugs, including alcohol and prescription and illegal drugs.[49]

Another study, published in 2014, found that states that have legalized medical marijuana have, on average, a 25% lower rate of opioid overdose deaths. The study also concluded that the longer the laws have been in effect, the greater the reduction in overdose deaths.[50]

Legal Status of Medical Marijuana

As of November 2014, medical marijuana was legal in 23 states and the District of Columbia. The first state to approve medical marijuana was California in 1996.[51]

All uses of marijuana remain illegal under federal law. According to the federal Controlled Substances Act (CSA), passed in 1970, it is illegal to possess or sell marijuana for any purpose.[52] According to the CSA, marijuana is a classified as a Schedule I drug—a controlled substance with a high potential for abuse and no currently accepted medical use.[53] Federal law prohibits "dispensing" a controlled substance, which has been widely interpreted to include the writing of prescriptions by physicians.[54] As a result, few physicians are willing to risk their medical licenses by prescribing medical marijuana even in states that have legalized medical marijuana. And because it's also a federal crime for pharmacies to distribute it, patients cannot legally fill their marijuana prescriptions.[55]

In 2005, the US Supreme Court ruled that federal laws superseded state marijuana laws.[56] States that have passed medical marijuana laws have done so in defiance of federal law in the belief that medical marijuana can help alleviate suffering. [57]

Practically speaking, the federal government cannot require state law enforcement agents to enforce federal laws, and few drug arrests are carried out by federal agents in states where medical marijuana is legal because of limited resources. As a result, arrests and prosecutions of doctors and patients for medical marijuana in states with medical marijuana laws are rare.[58]

The Case of Valery Corral

The federal Drug Enforcement Agency (DEA) has, however, focused on medical marijuana dispensaries in its efforts to curtail the use of medical marijuana. In one particularly onerous example, in 2002, 20 to 30 armed DEA agents appeared with a search warrant at a farm that grew medical marijuana for a California hospice. The 250 hospice patients suffered from AIDS, multiple sclerosis, cancer, and other terminal illnesses. Valery Corral, the owner of the farm, also owned the hospice and was herself a medical marijuana patient. The DEA agents entered the farm premises by force, pointed loaded firearms at Valery Corral and her husband, forced them onto the ground, and then handcuffed them. The Corrals were brought to the federal courthouse in San Jose and then released without being charged. DEA agents seized 167 marijuana plants that were the hospice patients' weekly supply of medication, which resulted in an increase of pain and suffering for the affected patients and hastened the death of some of them. All the hospice patients were prescribed medical marijuana by their physicians in accordance with local laws. In a subsequent court case challenging the federal action, as in all other cases involving medical marijuana dispensaries, the federal law was upheld.[59]

Changing Attitudes Toward Medical Marijuana

In 2007, the DEA sent letters to owners of buildings that housed medical marijuana dispensaries in California, threatening to charge them with felonies, seize their property and other assets, and send them to prison for up to 20 years. These threats resulted in the closure of more dispensaries.[60] The DEA has also raided medical marijuana dispensaries in other states.[61]

As part of a federal spending bill passed by congress and signed by President Obama on December 16, 2014, federal agents are now prohibited from raiding medical marijuana dispensaries in states that have legalized medical marijuana.[62]

In 2008, the American College of Physicians (ACP), the second largest physician group in the United States, released a position paper on medical marijuana. The paper urged that marijuana be reclassified into a more appropriate schedule, given the evidence of marijuana's safety and effectiveness in treating many clinical conditions. The paper also called for legally protecting physician's rights to prescribe medical marijuana and patients' rights to use marijuana without threat of prosecution, as allowed by state law. The paper included 10 pages of scientific documentation and references supporting its position. Former Surgeon General Jocelyn Elders endorsed the ACP's position.[63]

A 2011 poll of US adults by CBS News found that 77% agreed that doctors should be allowed to prescribe marijuana for serious illnesses.[64] An international poll of physicians in 2013 conducted by the *New England Journal of Medicine* found that 76% were in favor of medical use of marijuana.[65]

Joe

Like countless other chronic pain sufferers, Joe uses marijuana illicitly to relieve his suffering. Now 63 years old, Joe has been in pain for more than 20 years. His pain started when he hurt his back after crashing his car into a tree. Subsequent to that, he developed hand, elbow, wrist, and knee pain.

Joe (cont.)

About five or six years ago, he developed neuropathy of unknown origin. Despite his widespread pain, Joe worked at a physically demanding job until a couple of years ago, when he was laid off. He managed his pain with ibuprofen, Tylenol, or prescription drugs throughout the years until gastrointestinal side effects of the drugs became intolerable.

While Joe had used marijuana recreationally when he was younger, he had not used it for some time. Then, about a year ago, Joe's adult son visited and brought some marijuana, which they smoked together. After that, Joe discovered that his pain was much better for a couple of hours.

Since that time, Joe has smoked marijuana, which he acquires from friends, every evening to get some respite from his suffering. He doesn't use it during the day, when his wife, who also has numerous health problems, is out of the home, in case she needs him to pick her up. He said that about 1/8 of a teaspoon, smoked in a pipe, will do the trick. He estimates his marijuana "habit" costs him only about $50 a year because he uses such small amounts.

Joe's marijuana use is not without repercussions, however. Joe lives in upstate New York, where medical marijuana is still illegal. Although New York State passed a medical marijuana law in 2014, it does not take effect until 2016 and even then will not allow medical marijuana to be dispensed in a form that can be smoked—even though smoking is much more effective for pain relief than oral ingestion. Joe says he has been reluctant to look for another job for fear of being drug tested. That fear, more than the pain, keeps him from seeking employment.

A 2015 decision by the Colorado Supreme Court upheld an employer's right to fire an employee for using marijuana for medical purposes, even in states where medical marijuana is legal and the use is off-duty.[66]

Increasing Cannabinoids Without Marijuana

If you would like to increase your supply of cannabinoids without using marijuana, research suggests that exercise increases the body's supply of endocannabinoids. Studies have shown that moderate endurance exercise increases concentrations of anandamide, a natural cannabinoid, in blood plasma. This may be the mechanism behind the analgesic, stress-relieving, and mood-elevating effects of exercise.[67]

CHAPTER 14
LOW LEVEL LASER THERAPY

Low level laser therapy (LLLT) has been in use in Europe as a medical treatment for more than 40 years. Only recently has it begun attracting significant interest in the United States.

Two types of lasers are used for medical purposes. High power lasers are used to cut through tissue; low level lasers have the opposite effect—they stimulate tissue repair. In LLLT, a light is applied to an area of the body to relieve pain, reduce inflammation, and promote tissue regeneration. The light is usually a laser or LED between 1 mW and 550 mW in the red or near infrared spectrum. It's typically applied to the injured area for a very short time, generally a minute or so, a few times a week for a few weeks. The effect has been compared to photosynthesis, in which the absorbed light causes a chemical change in the tissue.[1]

The process by which low level lasers promote healing is called photomodulation. Three levels of effects have been identified.

1. Primary tissue effects are direct chemical effects on cells. LLLT increases the production of adenosine triphosphate (ATP), the fuel our cells use for energy. The more ATP available to our cells, the faster we heal. LLLT also increases the permeability of cell membranes, which allows waste products to be removed and nutrition to be absorbed into the cells more efficiently.

2. Secondary effects are chemical chain reactions that occur in response to the changes in the cells. LLLT secondary effects include anti-inflammatory effects, decreases in nerve irritability, and an increase in circulation in the area of injury or chronic pain.

3. Tertiary effects are whole-body effects from the treatment and include increased immune cell production, increased production of endorphins (the body's own painkillers), and improved nerve function.

Research Results

The process whereby low level lasers can stimulate growth was discovered in 1967, soon after the first laser was invented. As of 2009, more than 100 large randomized double-blind placebo-controlled human studies of LLLT had been published worldwide, as well as more than 1,000 scientific studies investigating the underlying mechanisms that contribute to its local and systemic effects.

Positive results have been reported for a very broad range of conditions, including the following:

- Osteoarthritis
- Tendonitis
- Wound healing
- Back and neck pain
- Muscle fatigue
- Peripheral nerve injuries
- Traumatic brain injuries
- Spinal cord injuries
- Stroke[2]
- Postherpetic neuralgia.[3]

The potential of LLLT continues to interest the medical research community, as indicated by the continued acceleration in the number of studies published. In just the last six years the number of studies has quadrupled, with 400 LLLT randomized clinical trials and more than 4,000 laboratory studies published.[4] Most, but not all, studies have been positive. The negative study results have been attributed to many factors related to less than optimum application of the LLLT, including too high or too low a dose or treating insufficient or inappropriate areas, as well as use by the patient of medications such as steroids or NSAIDs that can interfere with healing.[5,6]

A 2010 systematic review and meta-analysis of 16 randomized controlled trials of LLLT for the treatment of acute and chronic neck pain published in *Lancet* found that LLLT reduces pain immediately after treatment for acute injuries and for up to 22 weeks (the longest follow-up period of any of the studies) in patients with chronic neck pain. Patients received an average of 10 treatments. Side effects were the same as in the placebo groups.[7]

A 2010 meta-analyses of 22 studies published in the *Clinical Journal of Pain* investigated the magnitude of relief experienced by patients receiving LLLT for a variety of chronic pain conditions. A statistically significant and large effect was found.[8]

A 2015 review and meta-analysis of LLLT for shoulder tendon injuries (tendinopathy) evaluated 17 randomized controlled clinical trials. Reviewers found that LLLT resulted in significant "clinically relevant" improvements in pain and speeded recovery, either when provided alone or in combination with physical therapy interventions.[9]

A 2015 meta-analysis reviewed 49 randomized controlled trials of laser acupuncture, which uses low level laser at acupuncture points, for treatment of musculoskeletal disorders. The reviewers found that 31 of the studies were of high methodological quality and reported the dose adequately. These studies were uniformly positive. Poor-quality studies that did not provide dosage information tended to have negative or inconclusive results. The reviewers also reported that the positive effects were seen at long-term follow-up rather than immediately after treatment.[10]

A 2015 review and meta-analysis of LLLT in the treatment of temporomandibular disorders (TMDs), which are disorders of the jaw muscles, evaluated 14 randomized controlled trials. Reviewers found that LLLT did not improve pain levels compared to placebo, but treated patients had improved range of motion in their jaw that improved function.[11]

A 2015 study reported on a five-year follow-up of 50 back pain patients who had discography (a procedure to confirm that an abnormal disc was generating the pain) and who then were treated with LLLT. The patients received three LLLT sessions per week for 12 weeks. Forty-nine patients had significant improvement on a scale that measures disability at the end of the course of treatment. The improvements were found to be maintained at one-year and five-year follow-ups.[12]

A 2006 study reviewed the medical records of 2,239 patients, mean age 73, with peripheral neuropathy who had loss of sensation and neuropathic pain. After being treated with monochromatic infrared photo energy (MIRE), a low level laser therapy, there was an average improvement of 66%; 53% of the patients had fully regained sensation. In the patients with neuropathic pain, there was a 67% reduction in pain.[13]

Another study the same year with MIRE-treated patients, mean age 76, with diabetic neuropathy found that the symptomatic improvement gained from the treatment reduced falls by 78%, reduced balance-related fear of falling by 79%, and increased activities of daily living by 72% in the following year.[14]

LLLT treatment is generally regarded as safe. Many suggest LLLT is contraindicated for direct treatment of cancerous tumors or direct treatment of the thyroid because of its cell growth-stimulating effects, though there are some studies that show a positive effect even in these conditions.[15]

James Carroll, Thor Photomedicine CEO

James Carroll has been a man on a mission since 1988, when he first heard about LLLT. At the time, Carroll was in business helping companies raise grant money. One company he was advising was making lasers. The chief scientist there was reporting "amazing" results. Carroll thought the technology would be in widespread use all over the world within five years. He went to work for the laser company and soon after started his own company.

Carroll is disappointed but not deterred by the fact that the technology has not caught on like wildfire as he had expected. He is based in the United Kingdom but travels all over the world promoting the technology, including the United States, Iran, Iraq, South Africa and Australia. He even spoke at the UN Global Health Impact Fund. His current goal is to have his devices in 100 countries, treating 100 pathologies, by the time he's 100 years old. Beyond that, he'd like to see LLLT devices in every doctor's office, every hospital, and every home.

Carroll reports that "medical mavericks" in 72 countries are currently using his company's devices. Thousands of LLLT devices have been purchased by doctors in the United Kingdom who work for the National Health Service (NHS). The only countries he knows of that officially cover it through health insurance are Norway and Denmark.

Carroll's company is creating some innovative devices. One, specifically, treats dry macular degeneration, the leading cause of blindness globally. Another is a tanning-bed-like device that can treat the whole body, to treat "creaky old people" as well as systemic disorders.[16]

Steven Pershing, MD

Dr. Steve Pershing, who practices internal medicine in Tennessee, reports that he first became interested in low level laser therapy for wound care when he was a consulting physician for nursing homes but was unable to convince the proprietors to purchase LLLT devices. He then established a private practice and began using LLLT for pain and other disorders. He became interested in alternative pain treatment modalities partly because there are more opioid overdose deaths in Tennessee than deaths from motor vehicle accidents. He has been using LLLT for two years to treat a wide variety of conditions, including diabetic ulcers, musculoskeletal injuries, postsurgical healing, plantar fasciitis, gout, and lupus. He often sees dramatic results, even in one or two sessions. Pershing treated himself with the device when he had to have abdominal surgery. He used it pre- and post-surgery and had minimal pain and no inflammation. His doctor offered him pain medication, but he said no thanks, he didn't need it.

Pershing provided the following case histories:

Ginny

Ginny is the mother of a successful chiropractor. Her son was unable to help her with her spondylosis, a degeneration of the disc spaces between the vertebrae, which had advanced to the point that Ginny was tilted forward as she walked. After two LLLT treatments she was walking upright. She was treated twice a week for a month to resolve her pain. She now receives once a month maintenance treatment.

Ben

Ben was a long term diabetic who had numerous complications from the disease. He had already lost some toes to amputation. He had a very large ulcer on the back of his leg that wouldn't heal. The ulcer was a year old and Ben had already had skin grafts that had failed. Another doctor recommend-ed another skin graft. Pershing suggested that he try the LLLT instead. Within two months the wound had completely healed over. After six months the skin started to break down again. Ben was again treated with LLLT with rapid improvement.

Jason

Jason was a star high school basketball player with a college scholarship in hand when he suffered a severe high ankle sprain. These types of sprains generally take six weeks to heal. Jason was injured on a Saturday and treated the following Monday with LLLT. By Thursday he was able to walk around and a week later he was back to playing basketball

I was so impressed with what I was hearing about LLLT that I decided to order a system for my personal use from Thor. The salesperson, Valerie Gause, told me her own story:

Valerie

Valerie had suffered numerous whiplash-type injuries. As a young girl growing up she rode horses and fell off her horses repeatedly. She also had two car accidents--a rollover accident and an accident that involved a crash in an intersection when she wasn't wearing a seat belt.

Valerie (cont.)

She managed her neck pain with chiropractic, massage and self-care. In 2007 she heard about laser therapy from a dentist she spoke with in an airport but she dismissed him as a quack. Two years later Valerie had an exacerbation of her neck injury that became so severe that she couldn't lift her arm unless she lifted it with her other arm. Nothing worked and after 5 weeks her chiropractor suggested surgery. Valerie was uninsured at the time and couldn't afford surgery. Then she remembered what the dentist had told her about LLLT. After 3 LLLT treatments she felt fine.

FDA Approved but Unreimbursed

LLLT medical devices are FDA approved for "the temporary relief of pain." According to the FDA's website, this approval was based on "the presentation of clinical data to support such claims".[17] Despite this, and the extraordinary body of scientific evidence available on safety and effectiveness, most US insurance companies[18,19,20,] and Medicare[21] claim LLLT is investigational, experimental, or unproven and refuse to pay for this treatment for any condition.

CHAPTER 15

MULTIDISCIPLINARY PROGRAMS

According to the International Association for the Study of Pain (IASP), "Of all approaches to the treatment of chronic pain, none has a stronger evidence basis for efficacy, cost-effectiveness, and lack of iatrogenic [treatment-induced] complications than interdisciplinary care."[1]

By the 1980s, many hospitals in the United States had set up multidisciplinary pain programs. Patients were weaned off narcotics and other drugs and then put through a program that included medication management, graded physical exercise, and cognitive and behavioral techniques for pain and stress management. Biofeedback was also included in many programs.

A 1992 review of 65 studies found that multidisciplinary treatments were superior to single-discipline treatments, such as medical treatment or physical therapy, for chronic back pain. The review also found that the effects were stable over time and resulted in improvements in pain and mood, a greater likelihood of return to work, and lowered use of the health care system.[2]

A systematic review of 10 studies of multidisciplinary pain management programs published in the *British Medical Journal* in 2001 found that intensive (greater than 100 hours of therapy) multidisciplinary biopsychosocial rehabilitation programs produced greater reduction in pain and improvement in function for patients with disabling low-back pain than less-intensive multidisciplinary or non-multidisciplinary rehabilitation or usual care.[3] A 2004 follow-up study found that patients who had completed a multidisciplinary chronic pain program 13 years earlier had maintained their treatment gains from the program in all areas, including pain intensity, pain interference with daily functioning, and mood. The majority were employed, and few of the ones who were not reported that it was because of pain.[4]

With the introduction of OxyContin and other powerful opioids, insurers saw pills as a cheaper way of treating pain and, by 2000, had stopped funding these multidisciplinary programs.[5] The number of accredited multidisciplinary pain management programs in the United States decreased from more than 1,000 in 1999[6] to about 150 in 2011, with 49 of those programs accessible only to veterans.[7] That translates to one multidisciplinary pain clinic for every 3,244,444 nonveteran Americans, more than 33% of whom are in chronic pain. According to a survey by the International Association for the Study of Pain, published in 2012, the availability of this type of care worldwide (Europe, Canada, Australia, New Zealand, Israel) has been steadily increasing in the last decade everywhere except in the United States, with the exception of the VA Medical System.[8]

In 1995, the average cost of a multidisciplinary pain management program in the United States was estimated at $15,339.[9] In contrast, a conservative estimate of the cost of back surgery in 1997 was $27,577 per operation,[10] and the five-year cost estimate for a surgically implanted spinal cord stimulator after a failed back surgery was $144,255.[11]

According to a 2011 comprehensive report by the US Institute of Medicine, *Relieving Pain in America: A Blueprint for Transforming Prevention, Care, Education, and Research*:

Interdisciplinary, biopsychosocial approaches are the most promising for treating patients with persistent pain. But for most patients [and clinicians], such care is a difficult to attain ideal, impeded by numerous structural barriers— institutional, educational, organizational, and reimbursement related. Costly procedures often are performed when other actions should be considered, such as prevention, counseling, and facilitation of self-care, which are common features of successful treatment.[12]

Given the lack of integrated pain management programs, pain patients must find their own way through a complicated maze of treatment options to cobble together a program that might work for them. Most of the more effective and safer options are not covered by their insurance.

CHAPTER 16

THE PAIN TREATMENT PARITY ACT:

ONE PROPOSAL TO CURB TWO EPIDEMICS

Two devastating epidemics are raging across America: chronic pain, which affects 116 million Americans, and opioid abuse and addiction, which has 2 million Americans in its grip, with tens of thousands dying annually of opioid overdoses.

These two epidemics are causally related. A monumental increase in the number of opioid prescriptions written for chronic pain patients has resulted in a huge increase in the number of medical users and those who steal from their medicine cabinets becoming addicted to prescription opioids. When they can no longer get adequate amounts of the opioids from legitimate channels, they turn to heroin on the street, which is cheaper and more readily available than prescription painkillers.

Although many are calling for tighter monitoring of prescription painkillers, to date these efforts have only pushed those addicted into using heroin instead. Many others are calling for more drug treatment facilities to address the rising tide of addiction. While this response is necessary to care for those already hooked, it is not adequate to address the full problem. Drug treatment is costly, often ineffective, and occurs only after individuals, families, and communities have already suffered grave harm.

Preventing addiction is key. The best way to do this is to reduce the number of new prescriptions for opioids dispensed to chronic pain patients. Fortunately, curtailing opioid prescriptions can be done without harming pain patients, because safer, more effective pain treatments exist.

However, there are significant barriers to accessing the alternative pain treatments. Financial obstacles due to lack of insurance coverage, inadequate availability of services, and lack of knowledge of alternatives by both patients and their physicians prevent patients from receiving the most appropriate care.

A significant factor that has led to inadequate availability of many pain treatments is the fact that nonphysician in-network treatment providers, who are currently reimbursed for some care, have not, for the most part, received any fee increases in more than 35 years, whereas physician providers have received numerous increases. These nonphysician providers include chiropractors, physical therapists, occupational therapists, and mental health treatment providers. Availability of services has decreased as more providers are leaving their respective fields and fewer providers are entering these disciplines because of a 65% decline in real wages owing to inflation.[1]

The Pain Treatment Parity Act

To reduce these impediments to effective pain treatment and address these dual epidemics, I propose a Pain Treatment Parity Act (PTPA). The PTPA is loosely modeled after the Paul Wellstone and Pete Domenici Mental Health Parity and Addiction Equity Act of 2008 (MHPAEA), a federal law that prevents health insurance companies that provide mental health or substance use disorder benefits from imposing less-favorable benefit limitations on those benefits than on medical/surgical benefits.

The Pain Treatment Parity Act would require all entities that pay for treatment of chronic pain—including public and private health insurers (commercial insurers, HMOs, Medicare, and Medicaid); workers' compensation insurers; and automobile insurers—to cover all pain treatments that have credible evidence of effectiveness to the same degree that they cover pharmaceutical treatment of pain. This includes both qualitative and quantitative limitations on care, such as equivalence in pretreatment authorization requirements, limits on number of visits or dosage restrictions, co-payment requirements, as well as equivalent fee schedules.

Provisions of the PTPA

1. All pain treatments with some credible evidence of effectiveness must be covered when provided by a licensed or certified provider. This includes any treatments with at least one well-designed randomized, controlled trial showing a significant benefit from the therapy and a good safety profile or any other reasonable evidence of safety and effectiveness. Therapies that currently meet this standard include chiropractic, physical and occupational therapy, acupuncture, biofeedback, massage therapy, homeopathy, nutritional counseling and supplements, herbal therapy, psychotherapy, energy medicine therapy, supervised exercise programs, low level laser therapy, and multidisciplinary interventions, including coordination of services.

2. There can be no restrictions on the number of treatment visits or length of treatment for nonpharmaceutical pain treatment unless there are similar restrictions on dosage or length of treatment for the preponderance of pharmaceutical treatments for pain.

3. Co-pays for visits to nonphysician pain treatment providers cannot exceed the co-payment for primary care physician visits.

4. There cannot be a separate deductible for nonphysician pain treatment providers.

5. Preauthorization for visits to nonphysician pain treatment providers cannot be required unless preauthorization is required for the preponderance of pharmaceutical treatments for pain.

6. Medical necessity reviews cannot occur with greater frequency for nonphysician pain treatment providers than for physicians who provide pharmaceutical treatment for pain.

7. Fee schedules for in-network chiropractors, physical therapists, occupational therapists, psychologists, social workers, mental health counselors, acupuncturists, massage therapists, and all other nonphysician pain treatment providers must be increased by the same percentage as the average increase in fees for physicians for all specialties since 1980.

8. If an insurance plan has out-of-network benefits for medical and surgical treatments, it must also cover nonphysician out-of-network pain care providers at the same level of reimbursement.

9. All medical schools must offer a required course in pain management that educates students about all currently available treatments and the body of evidence supporting their use.

10. All physicians who treat chronic pain patients who have not completed a course in pain management in medical school must complete a 12-hour continuing medical education course about the safety and efficacy of all currently available treatments for chronic pain.

The Pain Treatment Parity Coalition

I am in the process of forming a coalition of health care providers, national and state health care provider associations, patients, policymakers, and other interested organizations and individuals to advocate at the state and federal levels for the PTPA. If you are willing and able to support this effort in any way, including administrative support or financial donations, please contact me at cindyperlin@gmail.com. Put "PTPA" in the subject line of your email.

Notes

Introduction (pp. 1–6)

[1] Institute of Medicine Report from the Committee on Advancing Pain Research, Care, and Education. (2011) *Relieving Pain in America, a Blueprint for Transforming Prevention, Care, Education and Research.* Washington, D.C.: The National Academies Press.

[2] *Global Industry Analysts, Inc. Report.* (2011) Retrieved from http://www.prweb.com/pdfdownload/8052240.pdf.

[3] National Centers for Health Statistics. *Chartbook on Trends in the Health of Americans 2006, Special Feature: Pain.* Retrieved from http://www.cdc.gov/nchs/data/hus/hus06.pdf.

[4] Al Mazroa, M.A. (2012) Years lived with disability (YLDs) for 1160 sequelae of 289 diseases and injuries 1990-2010: A systematic analysis for the Global Burden of Disease Study 2010. *Lancet, 380*(9859), 2163-96.

[5] Institute of Medicine. (2011). *Relieving Pain in America.*

[6] Tang, N. K., & Crane C. (2006). Suicidality in chronic pain: a review of the prevalence, risk factors and psychological links. *Psychological Medicine, 36*(5), 575-86.

[7] Torrance, N., Elliott, A., Lee, A., & Smith, B. (2010) Severe chronic pain is associated with increased 10 year mortality: A cohort record linkage study. *European Journal of Pain, 14*(4), 380–86.

[8] Institute of Medicine. (2011). *Relieving Pain in America.*

[9] International Association for the Study of Pain. Classification of chronic pain: Descriptions of chronic pain syndromes and definitions of pain terms. Prepared by the International Association for the Study of Pain, Subcommittee on Taxonomy. Pain Suppl S1–S226, 1986.

[10] American Academy of Pain Management. Facts on Pain. Retrieved from http://www.painmed.org/patientcenter/facts_on_pain.aspx#overview.

[11] Mezei L., Murinson B. & the Johns Hopkins Pain Curriculum Development Team. (2011) Pain education in North American schools. *The Journal of Pain, 12*(12),1199-1208.

[12] Based on a survey of tables of contents by my research assistant, Beth Eisman.

[13] Based on a survey of conference offerings by my research assistant, Beth Eisman.

[14] American Academy of Pain Management: Members. Retrieved from ttp://www.aapainmanage.org/membership/.

[15] O'Rorke J. E., Chen I., Genao M., & Cykert S. (2007). Physicians comfort in caring for patients with chronic nonmalignant pain. *American Journal of Medical Sciences, 333*(2),93-100.

[16] Green C. R. (2003). Physician variability in the management of acute postoperative and cancer pain: A quantitative assessment of the Michigan Experience. *Pain Medicine, 4,* 8-20.

[17] Upshur C., Bacigalupe G., & Luckmann R. "They don't want anything to do with you": Patient views of primary care management of chronic pain. *Pain Medicine 2010; 11:1791-1798.*

Chp. 1: How Do We Know What Works (pp. 7–16)

[1] Sackett D. L., Rosenberg W. M. C., Gray J. A. M., Haynes R. B., & Richardson, W. S. (1996) Evidence based medicine: What it is and what it isn't. *The BMJ, 312,* 71-2.

[2] U.S. Agency for Health Care Policy and Research guidelines

[3] Every-Palmer, S. & Howick, J. (2014) How evidence-based medicine is failing due to biased trials and selective publication. *Journal of Evaluation in Clinical Practice, 20,* 908-14.

[4] Ioannidis, J. P. (2008) Effectiveness of antidepressants: an evidence myth constructed from a thousand randomized trials? *Philosophy, Ethics and Humanities in Medicine, 3,* 14.

[5] CBI Research. (2012) Antidepressants market to 2018–Despite safety concerns, selective serotonin re-uptake inhibitors (SSRIs) continue to dominate in the absence of effective therapeutic alternatives. http://www.gbiresearch.com/Report.aspx?ID=Antidepressants-Market-to-2018-Despite-Safety-Concerns

-Selective-Serotonin-Re-uptake-Inhibitors-(SSRIs)-Continue-to-Dominate-in-the-Absence-of-Effective-Therapeutic-Alternatives.

[6] Kirsch, I., Deacon, B. J., Huedo-Medina, T. B., Scoboria, A., Moore, T. J. & Johnson, B. T. (2008) Initial severity and antidepressant benefits: a meta-analysis of data submitted to the food and drug

administration. *PLoS Medicine, 5,* e45.

[7] Fournier, J. C., DeRubeis, R. J., Hollon, S. D., Dimidjian, S., Amsterdam, J. D., Shelton, R. C. & Fawcett, J. (2010). Antidepressant drug effects and depression severity: A patient level meta-analysis. *Journal of the American Medical Association, 303,* 47–53.

[8] Heres, S., Davis, J., Maino, K., Jetzinger, E., Kissling,W. & Leucht, S. (2006). Why olanzapine beats risperidone, risperidone beats quetiapine, and quetiapine beats olanzapine: an exploratory analysis of head-to-head comparison studies of second-generation antipsychotics. *American Journal of Psychiatry, 163,*185–94.

[9] Smith, R. (2005) Medical journals are an extension of the marketing arm of pharmaceutical companies. *PLoS Medicine,* 2 (5), e138.

[10] Shellenberger, R. and Green, J. A. (1986). *From the Ghost in the Box to Successful Biofeedback Training.* Greely, CO: Health Psychology Publications.

[11] Shellenberger & Green. (1986). *From the Ghost in the Box to Successful Biofeedback Training.*

[12] Banderia, M., Bouchard, M., & Granger L. Voluntary control of autonomic responses: A case for a dialogue between individual and group experimental methodolgies. *Biofeedback and Self-Regulation, 7,* 317-329.

[13] Shellenberger & Green. (1986). *From the Ghost in the Box,* 15-64.

[14] Roehr, B. (2012). GlaxoSmithKline is fined record $3 billion in US. *British Medical Journal, 345,* e4568.

[15] Lenzer, J. (2006). Manufacturer admits increase in suicidal behaviour in patients taking paroxetine. *British Medical Journal, 332*(7551), 1175.

[16] Department of Justice. (2012) GlaxoSmithKline to plead guilty and pay $3 billion to resolve fraud allegations and failure to report safety data. http://www.justice.gov/opa/pr/2012/July/12-civ-842.html.

[17] Kmietowicz, Z. (2012). Johnson & Johnson to pay $2.2 bn to settle charges of false marketing on three drugs. B*ritish Medical Journal, 347,* f6696.

[18] Tanne, J. H. (2012). US judge fines Johnson & Johnson $1.1 bn for misleading marketing of risperidone. *British Medical Journal, 344,* e2772.

[19] Tanne. (2012). US judge fines Johnson & Johnson.

[20] Borrell, B. (2009, March 10). A medical Madoff: Anesthesiologist faked data in 21 studies. *Scientific American,*

[21] Press release, FDA Office of Criminal Investigations/US Department of Justice. Anesthesiologist sentenced on health care fraud charge, June 24, 2010. http://www.fda.gov/ICECI/CriminalInvestigations/ucm217302.ht m on 8/10/15.

[22] Borrell. (2009). A medical Madoff.

[23] Every-Palmer & Howick. (2014). How evidence-based medicine is failing.

[24] Researching Integrative Medicine: Challenges and Innovations available at http://exploreim.ucla.edu/research/researching-integrative-medicine-challenges-and-innovations/#funding

[25] Hartzband, P. & Groopman, J. (2014, November 18). How medical care is being corrupted. *New York Times,*

[26] Shellenberger & Green. (1986). *From the Ghost in the Box.*

[27] Shellenberger & Green. (1986). *From the Ghost in the Box.*

[28] Van der Kolk, Bessel. (2015). Workshop presentation at the Cape Cod Institute.

[29] Personal interview.

Chp. 2: Pharmaceutical Treatments (pp. 17–42)

[1] Manchikanti, L. & Singh A. (2008). Therapeutic Opioids: A Ten-Year Perspective on the Complexities and Complications of the Escalating Use, Abuse, and Nonmedical Use of Opioids. *Pain Physician 2008: Opioids Special Issue, 11*:S64-S88.

[2] Manchikanti & Singh. (2008). Therapeutic Opioids.

[3] Manchikanit & Singh. (2008). Therapeutic Opioids, S80.

[4] Trescot, A., Glaser, S., Hansen, H., Benyamin, R., Patel, S., & Manchikanti, L. (2008). Effectiveness of Opioids in the Treatment of Chronic Non-Cancer Pain, *Pain Physician 2008: Opioids Special Issue: 11*, S181-S200.

[5] Manchikanti & Singh. (2008). Therapeutic Opioids. p.S80.

[6] Vogt, M. T., Kwoh C. K., Cope, D. K., Osial, T. A., Culyba, M., & Starz,

T. W. (2005). Analgesic usage for low-back pain: Impact on health care costs and service use. *Spine, 30*, 1075-81.

[7] Webster, B. S., Verma, S. K., & Gatchel, R. J. (2007). Relationship between early opioid prescribing for acute occupational low-back pain and disability duration, medical costs, subsequent surgery, and late opioid use. *Spine, 32*, 2127-2132.

[8] Mahmud M. A., Webster, B. S., Courtney, T. K., Matz, S., Tacci, J. A., & Christiani D. C. (2000). Clinical management and the duration of disability for work-related low-back pain. *JOccup Environ Med, 42*, 1178-1187.

[9] Webster et al. (2007). Relationship between early opioid prescribing.

[10] Eriksen, J., Sjogren, P., Bruera, E., Ekholm, O., & Rasmussen, N. K. (2006). Critical issues on opioids in chronic non-cancer pain: An epidemiological study. *Pain, 125,*172-79.

[11] Chaparro, L. E., Furlan, A. D., Deshpande, A., Mailis-Gagnon, A., Atlas, S., & Turk, D. C.(2013). Opioids compared to other treatments for chronic low-back pain. *Cochrane Database Systematic Reviews, 8.*

[12] Prescription Painkiller Overdoses in the United States. (2011). *CDC Vital Signs.* http://www.cdc.gov/vitalsigns/PainkillerOverdoses/index.html.

[13] Prescription Painkiller Overdoses.

[14] Prescription Painkiller Overdoses.

[15] Prescription Painkiller Overdoses.

[16] Rosenblum, A., Joseph, H., Fong, C., et al. (2003.) Prevalence and characteristics of chronic pain among chemically dependent patients in methadone maintenance and residential treatment facilities. *JAMA, 289*(18), 2370-8.

[17] Hall, A. J., Logan, J. E., Toblin, R. L., et al. (2008). Patterns of abuse among unintentional pharmaceutical overdose fatalities. *JAMA, 300*, 2613-20.

[18] Martell, B., O'Connor, P., & Kerns, R. (2007). Systemic review: Opioid treatment for chronic back pain: Prevalence, efficacy, and association with addiction. *Annals of Internal Medicine, 146*(2), 116-27.

[19] Whoriskey, P. (2012. December 30). Rising painkiller addiction shows damage from drugmakers' role in shaping medical opinion. *The*

Washington Post.

[20] Eban, K. (2011, November 9). OxyContin: Purdue Pharma's painful medicine. *Fortune.* http://fortune.com/2011/11/09/oxycontin-purdue-pharmas-painful-medicine/

[21] Eban. (2011). OxyContin: Purdue Pharma's painful medicine.

[22] Eban, K., (2011, November 9). OxyContin: Purdue Pharma's painful medicine, *CNNMoney.* http://features.blogs.fortune.cnn.com/2011/11/09/oxycontin-purdue-pharma/.

[23] Hwang, C., Turner, L., Kruszewski, S., Kolodny, A., & Alexander, G. C. (2015). Primary care physicians' knowledge and attitudes regarding prescription opioid abuse and diversion. *The Clinical Journal of Pain.* [Epub ahead of print]

[24] Taraborrelli, J.R.(2009, June 29). 'I saw in his eyes he was dying': Michael Jackson's life-long confidante J. Randy Taraborrelli tells the real story of star's fall. *Daily Mail.*

[25] Macfarlane J. (2009, June 27). Michael Jackson's drugs cocktail 'was unusual and dangerous'. *Daily Mail.*

[26] Gottlieb, J. (2013, May 17) Michael Jackson Trial: Conrad Murray's payment demands 'outrageous'. *Los Angeles Times.*

[27] Barron, J. (2008, February 7). Medical examiner rules Ledger's death accidental. *New York Times.*

[28] Goodman, J.D. (2014, February 3). Hoffman's heroin points to surge in grim trade. *New York Times.*

[29] Bailey, J., Hurley, R., & Gold, M. (2010). Review article: Crossroads of Pain and Addiction, *Pain Medicine, 11,* 1803.

[30] Bailey, Hurley, & Gold. (2010). 1805.

[31] Gardner, E. (2008). Pain management and the so called risk of addiction: A neurobiological perspective. In *Pain and Chemical Dependency.* New York: New York University Press.

[32] Carey, B. (2014, February 10) Prescription painkillers seen as a gateway to heroin. *New York Times.*

[33] *NPR,* February 4, 2014. http://www.npr.org/2014/02/04/271591524/spike-in-heroin-use-can-be-traced-to-prescription-pads.

[34] Kosten, T. & George, T. (2002). The neurobiology of opioid dependence: implications for treatment. *Science and Practice Perspectives*, 13-20.

[35] Ramin, C. J. (2013). Why did the FDA approve a new pain drug? *The New Yorker*. http://www.newyorker.com/online/blogs/currency/2013/12/zohydro-why-did-the-fda-approve-a-new-pain-drug.html.

[36] Garbitelli, B. (2014, April24). States revolt against controversial new painkiller. *Huffington Post*. http://www.huffingtonpost.com/2014/04/04/zohydro-painkiller-states_n_5091103.html.

[37] Reuters. (2013, December 12). Staate AGs urge FDA to rethink approval of painkiller Zohydro. http://www.reuters.com/article/2013/12/12/us-usa-fda-zohydro-idUSBRE9BB1AQ20131212 on April 4, 2014.

[38] Glover, S. & Girion, L. (2014, May 21). Counties sue narcotics makers, alleging 'campaign of deception.' *Los Angeles Times*.

[39] Letter to Secretary Sylvia Mathews Burwell of the US Department of Health and Human Services by the Coalition to End the Opioid Epidemic, September 22, 2014, http://feduprally.org/wp-content/uploads/2014/09/Burwell-Letter-completed-with-signature-Final.pdf.

[40] CenterWatch Targiniq ER (oxycodone hydrochloride + naloxone hydrochloride) extended-release tablets. available at http://www.centerwatch.com/drug-information/fda-approved-drugs/drug/100018/targiniq-er-oxycodone-hydrochloride--naloxone-hydrochloride-extended-release-tablets.

[41] CenterWatch . Targiniq ER.

[42] Skilek, M., (2014, November 11). Bob Rapaport, MD, Division Director of Anesthesia, Analgesia and Addiction Products at FDA retires. *Salem News*. http://www.salem-news.com/articles/november112014/rappaport-retire-ms.php accessed on 11/16/14.

[43] Rabin, R. (2014, November 20). FDA approves Hysingla, a powerful painkiller. *The New York Times*.

[44] Wasserman, E. (2014, November 20). FDA approves Purdue's abuse-resistant Hysingla, a hydrocodone pill aimed at knocking off

Zohydro. *Fierce Pharma.*

[45] Bailey, Hurley, & Gold. (2010), 1804.

[46] Libby, R. (2008). *The Criminalization of Medicine: America's War on Doctors*, Wesport, Connecticut: Praeger, 119-125.

[47] Libby. *The Criminalization of Medicine*, 143-156.

[48] Vellejo, R., de Leon-Casasola, O., & Benyamin, R. (2004). Opioid therapy and immunosuppression. *American Journal of Therapeutics, 11*, 354-365.

[49] Whitten, L. (2008). Morphine-Induced immune suppression: from brain to spleen, National Institute of Drug Abuse. http://www.drugabuse.gov/news-events/nida-notes/2008/06/morphine-induced-immunosuppression-brain-to-spleen accessed on 12/23/12.

[50] Vellejo et al. (2004). Opioid therapy and immunosuppression.

[51] Sprouse-Blum, A.; Smith Gl Sugai, D., & Parsa, F.D. (2010). Understanding Endorphins and Their Importance in Pain Management, *Hawai'i Medical Journal, 69*, 70-71.

[52] Angst, M. & Clark, J.D. (2006). Opioid-induced hyperalgesia. *Anesthesiology, 104*, 570

[53] Angst & Clark. (2006). Opioid-induced hyperalgesia, 579.

[54] Angst & Clark. (2006). Opioid-induced hyperalgesia, 583.

[55] Gussenhover, R. (2014.) Chronic Pain, the opioid conundrum and pharmacy compounding. *The Pain Practitioner, 24*(2):43-45.

[56] National Institute of Drug Abuse. (2010). What is Drugged Driving. http://www.drugabuse.gov/publications/drugfacts/drugged-driving on 2/16/13.

[57] Prescription Painkiller Overdoses in the United States.(2011). *CDC Vital Signs.* http://www.cdc.gov/vitalsigns/PainkillerOverdoses/index.html on 11/23/12

[58] Mafi, J., McCarthy, E., Davis, R., & Landon, B. (2013). Worsening trends in the management and treatment of back pain. *JAMA Internal Medicine.*

[59] Glover, S. & Girion, L. Legal drugs, deadly outcomes. (2012, November 11). *Los Angeles Times.*

[60] Use of opioids for the treatment of chronic pain. (2014). PainMed. http://www.painmed.org/files/use-of-opioids-for-the-treatment-of-chronic-pain.pdf accessed on 6/16/14.

[61] Physicians for Responsible Opioid Prescribing. Cautious, evidence-based opioid prescribing. http://www.supportprop.org/educational/PROP_OpioidPrescribing .pdf accessed on 6/16/14

[62] Wikipedia. History of aspirin. http://en.wikipedia.org/wiki/History_of_aspirin accessed on 12/30/12.

[63] Wikipedia. History of aspirin. http://en.wikipedia.org/wiki/History_of_aspirin accessed on 12/30/12.

[64] FDA. Aspirin comprehensive prescribing information. http://www.fda.gov/ohrms/dockets/ac/03/briefing/4012B1_03_Ap pd%201-Professional%20Labeling.pdf accessed on 12/30/12

[65] Singh G. (2000) Gastrointestinal Complications of Prescription and over-the-counter nonsteroidal anti-inflammatory drugs: A view from the ARAMIS database. *American Journal of Therapeutics,* 7:115-121.

[66] Tavernise S. Experts urge sparing use of nonaspirin painkillers. *New York Times,* July 13, 2015

[67] U.S. National Library of Medicine. Ibuprofen. https://www.nlm.nih.gov/medlineplus/druginfo/meds/a682159.htm l

[68] Schiodt, F.V., Atillasoy, E., Shakil, A.O., et al. (1999). Etiology and outcome for 295 patients with acute liver failure in the United States. *Liver Transplant Surg, 5,* 29–34.

[69] McNeil Consumer & Specialty Pharmaceuticals. (2001). McNeil OTC habits & practices study. Data on file.

[70] Zimmerman, H.J. & Maddrey, W. C. (1995). Acetaminophen (paracetamol) hepatotoxicity with regular intake of alcohol: analysis of instances of therapeutic misadventure. *Hepatology, 22,* 767–3.

[71] Whitcomb, D. C. & Block, G. D. (1994). Association of acetaminophen hepatotoxicity with fasting and ethanol use. *JAMA, 272,* 1845–50.

[72] Good, P. (2009). Did Acetaminophen Provoke the Autism Epidemic? *Alternative Medicine Review, 14*(4).

[73] Bauer, A. & Kriebel, D. (2013). Prenatal and perinatal analgesic exposure and autism: an ecological link. *Environmental Health, 12,* 41.

[74] Bauer & Kriebel. (2013). Prenatal and perinatal analgesic exposure.

[75] Schultz, S. T., Klonoff-Cohen, H. S., Wingard, D. L., et al. (2008). Acetaminophen (paracetamol) use, measles-mumps-rubella vaccination, and autistic disorder: the results of a parent survey. *Autism, 12,* 293-307.

[76] Cockburn, A. (2012). When half a million Americans died and nobody noticed. *The Week.* http://www.theweek.co.uk/us/46535/when-half-million-americans-died-and-nobody-noticed on 11/15/14.

[77] http://www.drugwatch.com/vioxx/lawsuit/ accessed on 11/15/14.

[78] http://www.drugwatch.com/vioxx/lawsuit/ accessed on 11/15/14.

[79] http://www.drugwatch.com/vioxx/lawsuit/ accessed on 11/15/14.

[80] Thomas, K. (2012, June 24). In documents on Pain Drug, Signs of Doubt and Deception. *New York Times.*

[81] Thomas. (2012). In documents on Pain Drug.

[82] Caldwell, B., Aldington, S., Weatherall, M., Shirtcliffe, P., & Beasley, R. (2006). Risk of cardiovascular events and celecoxib: a systematic review and meta-analysis. *Journal of the Royal Society of Medicine, 99*(3),132-140.

[83] Thomas. (2012). In documents of Pain Drug.

[84] http://www.drugs.com/stats/celebrex accessed on 11/15/14.

[85] Treating Rheumatoid Arthritis. (2005, February). *Harvard Women's Health Watch,* 5.

[86] Vlad, S., et al. (2011). Short periods of glucocorticoid use are associated with a prolonged risk of osteonecrosis. American College of Rheumatology, Abstract 802.

[87] Department of Justice. (2004). Warner_ambert to pay $430 million to resolve criminal & civil health care liability relating to off-label promotion. http://www.justice.gov/archive/opa/pr/2004/May/04_civ_322.htm.

[88] Department of Justice. (2009). Justice department announces largest health care fraud settlement in its history. http://www.justice.gov/opa/pr/justice-department-announces-largest-health-care-fraud-settlement-its-history. Accessed on 11/16/14.

[89] Moore, R. A., Wiffen, P. J., Derry, S., Toelle, T., Andrew, S., & Rice, C. (2014). Gabapentin for chronic neuropathic pain and fibromyalgia in adults. *The Cochrane Library*.

[90] http://www.accessdata.fda.gov/drugsatfda_docs/label/2010/020235 s043lbl.pdf accessed on 11/16/14.

[91] http://1800theeagle.com/dangerous-drugs-news/2014/06/neurotonin-case-settled-pfizer/ accessed on 11/15/14.

[92] Antibiotics May Cure 40% of Chronic Back Pain Cases. (2013). *Medical News Today*. http://www.medicalnewstoday.com/articles/260274.php

Chp. 3: Injections for Pain (pp. 43–50)

[1] Bernstein, R. M. (2001). Injections and surgical therapy in chronic pain, *Clinical Journal of Pain, 17*(4 Suppl), S94-104.

[2] Scott, N. A., Guo, B., Barton, P. M., & Gerwin, R. D. (2009). Trigger Point Injections for Chronic Non-Malignant Musculoskeletal Pain: A Systematic Review, *Pain Medicine, 10*(1), 54-69.

[3] Radcliff, K., Kepler, C., Hilbrand, A., Rihn, J., Zhao, W., Lurie, J., Tosteson, T., Vaccar, A., Albert, T., & Weinstein, J. (2013). Epidural Steriod Injections Are Associated With Less Improvement in Patients With Spinal Stenosis: A Subgroup Analysis of the Spine Patients Outcomes Research Trial, *Spine, 38*(4), 279-291.

[4] Friedly, J., Comstock, B., Turner, J., Haegerty, P., Deyo, R., Sullivan, S., . . . & Jarvik JG. (2014). A randomized trial of epidural glucocorticoid injections for spinal stenosis. *New England Journal of Medicine, 371*(1),11-21.

[5] Bicket, M., Gupta, A., Brown, C., & Cohen, S. (2013). Epidural injections for spinal pain: A systematic review and meta-analysis evaluating the "control" injections in randomized controlled trials. *Anesthesiology, 119*(4), 907-931.

[6] Turk, D. C., Wilson, H. D., & Cahana, A. (2011). Pain 2: Treatment of

chronic non-cancer pain, *Lancet, 277*, 2230.

[7] http://www.fda.gov/Drugs/DrugSafety/ucm394280.htm accessed on 4/27/14.

[8] http://www.bcm.edu/news/item.cfm?newsID=6503 accessed on 2/16/13.

[9] Marcus, N. J., Gracely, E.J., & Keefe, K.O. (2010). A comprehensive protocol to diagnose and treat pain of muscular origin may successfully and reliably decrease or eliminate pain in a chronic pain population. *Pain Medicine, 11*, 25-34.

[10] Marcus, N. J., Shrikhande, A. A., McCarberg, B., & Gracely, E. (2013). A preliminary study to determine if a muscle pain protocol can produce long-term relief in chronic back pain patients. *Pain Medicine, 14*,1212-1221.

[11] Personal interview.

[12] According to the American College of Rheumatology, a diagnosis of fibromyalgia should be considered when a patient has at least 11 of 18 possible tender points that are painful under pressure.

Chp. 4: Surgical Treatments (pp. 51–59)

[1] Deyo, R.A. & Mirza, S.K. (2006). Trends and variations in the use of spine surgery. Clin Orthop Relat Res, *443*, 139–46.

[2] Cherkin, D. C., Deyo, R. A., Loeser, J. D., Bush, T., & Waddell, G. (1994). An international comparison of back surgery rates. *Spine, 19*, 1201–6.

[3] Keller, R. B., Atlas, S. J., Soule, D. N., Singer, D. E., & Deyo, R. (1999). Relationship between rates and outcomes of operative treatment of lumbar disc herniation and spinal stenosis. *J Bone Joint Surg Am*; *81*,752–62.

[4] Deyo, R. & Mirza, S. (2009). The case for restraint in spinal surgery: does quality management have a role to play? *European Spine Journal,18*(Suppl 3), S331-S337.

[5] Nachemson, A. (1993). Evaluation of results in lumbar spine surgery. *Acta Orthop Scand, 251*, 130–3.

[6] Chan, C. & Peng, P. (2011). Failed Back Surgery Syndrome. *Pain Medicine, 12*, 578.

[7] Burton CV. (2006). Failed back surgery patients: The alarm bells are ringing. *Surgical Neurology, 65*, 5–6.

[8] Peul, W. C., van Houwelingen, H. C., van den Hout, W. B., et al.; Leiden-The Hague Spine Intervention Prognostic Study Group. (2007). Surgery versus prolonged conservative treatment for sciatica. *New England Journal of Medicine, 356,* 2245–56.

[9] Peul, W. C., van den Hout, W. B., Brand, R., Thomeer, R. T. W. M., & Koes, B. W. (2008). Prolonged conservative care versus early surgery in patients with sciatica caused by lumbar disc herniation: Two year results of a randomized control trial. *British Medical Journal, 336,*1355–8.

[10] deKleuver, M., Oner, F. C., & Jacobs, W. C. (2003). Total disc replacement for chronic low-back pain: background and a systematic review of the literature. *European Spine Journal, 12*(2),108-16.

[11] Wilkinson, H. A. (1992). *The Failed Back Syndrome* (2nd ed.). New York: Springer-Verlag.

[12] de Lissovoy, G., Brown, R. E., Halpern, M., Hassenbusch, S. J., & Ross, E. (1997). Cost-effectiveness of long-term intrathecal morphine therapy for pain associated with failed back surgery syndrome. *Clin Ther, 19,* 96–112.

[13] Carragee, E. J., Alamin, T., Miller, J. L., & Carragee, J. M. (2005) Discographic, MRI and psychosocial determinants of low-back pain disability and remission: A prospective study in patients with benign back pain. *Spine Journal, 5,* 24–35.

[14] Celestin, J., Edwards, R. R., & Jamison, R. N. (2009). Pretreatment psychosocial variables as predictors of outcomes following lumbar surgery and spinal cord stimulation: A systematic review and literature synthesis. *Pain Medicine, 10,* 639–53.

[15] Mannion, A. F. & Elfering, A. (2006). Predictors of surgical outcome and their assessment. *European Spine Journal, 15,* S93–108.

[16] Bosacco, S. J., Berman, A. T., Bosacco, D. N., & Levenberg, R. J. (1995). Results of lumbar disc surgery in a city compensation population. *Orthopedics, 18,* 351–5.

[17] Klekamp, J., Mccarty, E., & Spengler, D. M. (1998). Results of elective lumbar discectomy for patients involved in the workers' compensation system. *Journal of Spinal Disorders, 11,* 277–82.

[18] Taylor, V. M., Deyo, R. A., & Ciol, M, et al. (2000). Patient-orientated outcomes from low back surgery: A communitybased study. *Spine,*

25, 2445–52.

[19] Waddell, G., Main, C. J., Morris, E. W., Di Paola, M., & Gray, I. C. M. (1984). Chronic low-back pain, psychologic distress, and illness behaviour. *Spine*, 9, 209–13.

[20] Schofferman, J., Anderson, D., Hines, R., Smith, G., & White, A. (1992). Childhood Psychological Trauma Correlates with Unsuccessful Lumbar Spine Surgery. *Spine*, *17*(6), S138-144.

[21] Grevitt, M., Pande, K., O'Dowd, J., & Webb, J.(1998). Do first impressions count? A comparison of subjective and psychological assessment of spinal patients. *European Spine*, 7, 218-223.

[22] Block, A., Ohnmeiss, D., Guyer, R., Rashbaum, R., & Hochschuler, S. (2001). The use of presurgical psychological screening to predict the outcome of spine surgery. *The Spine Journal, 1*(4), 274-282.

[23] Young, A. K.., Young, B. K., & Riley, L. H. 3rd. (2012). Skolasky Assessment of Psychological Screening in Patients Undergoing Spine Surgery, *Journal of Spinal Disorders and Techniques*.

[24] Committee on Finance United States Senate, (2012). Staff Report on Medtronic's Influence on Infuse Clinical Studies, 2-4. http://www.finance.senate.gov/newsroom/chairman/release/?id=b1 d112cb-230f-4c2e-ae55-13550074fe86

[25] Medtronic Surgeons Held Back, Study Said. (2011, June 29). *Wall Street Journal*.

[26] Medtronic Product Linked to Surgery Problems. (2008, September 4). *Wall Street Journal*.

[27] Data Links High Doses of Bone Drug to Cancer. (2011, November 3). *New York Times*.

[28] Data Links High Doses. (2011). *NYT*.

[29] Boden, S. D., Davis, D. O., Dina, T. S., Patronas, N. J., & Wiesel, S. W. (1990). Abnormal magnetic resonance scans of the lumbar spine in asymptomatic subjects: a prospective investigation. *Journal of Bone and Joint Surgery AM, 72*, 403-8.

[30] Jensen, M., Brant-Zawadzki, M., Obuchowski, N., Modic, M., Malkasian. D., & Ross, J. (1994). Magnetic resonance imaging of the lumbar spine in people without back pain. *New England Journal of Medicine, 331*(2), 69-72.

[31] Zimmerman, Robert D. (1997). A Review of Utilization of Diagnostic

Imaging in the Evaluation of Patients with Back Pain: The When and What of Back Pain Imaging. *Journal of Back and Musculoskeletal Rehabilitation, 8,* 125-33.

[32] Borenstein, G., Boden, S. D., Wiesel, S. W., et al. (2001). The value of magnetic resonance imaging of the lumbar spine to predict low-back pain in asymptomatic individuals: A 7-year follow-up study. *Journal of Bone and Joint* Surgery *AM, 83,* 320-34

[33] Boodman, S. (2014, May 26). For seven years, searing pain with no relief. *The Washington Post.*

[34] Smith, J. S., Sidhu, J., Bode, K., Gendelberg, D., Maltenfort, M., Ibrahimi, D., Shaffrey, C. I, Vaccaro, A. R. (2014). Operative and nonoperative treatment approaches for lumbar degenerative disc disease have similar long-term clinical outcomes among patients with positive discography. *World Neurosurgery , 82*(5), 872-878.

[35] Marcus, Norman, M. D. (2012). *End Back Pain Forever: A Groundbreaking Approach to Eliminate Your Suffering.* New York, Atria Books, 45.

[36] Marcus. *End of Back Pain Forever.* Atria.

[37] Marcus. *End of Back Pain Forever.* Atria.

[38] Moseley, J. & Bruce et al. (2002). A controlled trial of arthroscopic surgery for osteoarthritis of the knee. *New England Journal of Medicine, 347*(2), 81-88.

[39] Kirkly, A. et al. (2008). A randomized trial of arthroscopic surgery for osteoarthritis of the knee. *New England Journal of Medicine, 359*(22), 1097-1107.

[40] Kirkly, A. et al. (2008). A randomized trial of arthroscopic surgery for osteoarthritis of the knee. *New England Journal of Medicine, 359(*22), 1097-1107.

[41] Khan, M., Evaniew, N., Bedi, A,. Ayeni, O., & Bhandari, M. (2014). Arthroscopic surgery for degenerative tears of the meniscus: a systematic review and meta-analysis. *CMAJ* online. http://www.cmaj.ca/content/early/2014/08/25/cmaj.140433.full.pdf +html

[42] Mordecai, S. C., Al-Hadithy, N., Ware, H. E, & Gupte, C. M. (2014). Treatment of meniscal tears: An evidence based approach. *World Journal of Orthopedics, 5*(3)233-41.

[43] Mafi, J., McCarthy, E., Davis, R., & Landon, B. (2013). Worsening trends in the management and treatment of back pain, *JAMA Internal Medicine, 173*(170) 1573-1581.

Chp. 5: Mind/Body Treatments (pp. 61–86)

[1] Shubiner, H. (2012) *Unlearn Your Pain: A 28-Day Process to Reprogram Your Brain.* Pleasant Ridge, MI: Mind*Body Publishing.4.

[2] Shubiner. (2012). *Unlearn Your Pain.*

[3] Marcus, Norman, MD. (2012). *End Back Pain Forever: A Groundbreaking Approach to Eliminate Your Suffering.* New York, Atria Books, 67.

[4] Marcus. *End Back Pain Forever.* Atria, 66.

[5] Klossika, I., Flor, H., Kamping, S., et al.(2006). Emotional modulation of pain: A clinical perspective. *Pain, 124,* 264-268.

[6] Peyron, R., Laurent, M., & Garcie-Larria, L. (2000). Functional imaging of brain responses to pain: a review and meta-analysis. *Clinical Neurophysiology, 30,* 263-288.

[7] Leiberman, M. D., Jarco, J. M., Berman, S., Naliboff, B. D., Suyenobu, B. Y., Mandelkern, M., & Mayer, E A. (2004) The neural correlates of placebo effects: a disruption account. *Neuroimage, 22,* 447-455.

[8] Burns, J. W. (2006).Arousal of Negative emotions and symptom specific reactivity in chronic low-back pain patients. *Emotion, 6,* 309-19.

[9] Quartana, P. J. & Burns, J. W. (2007). Painful consequences of anger suppression. *Emotion, 7,* 400-14

[10] Burns, J, W., Qurtana, P. J., Matsuura, J., Gilliam, W., Nappi, C., & Wolfe, B. (2012). Suppression of anger and subsequent pain intensity and behavior among chronic low-back pain patients: the role of symptom-specific physiological reactivity. *Journal of Behavioral Medicine, 35*(1), 103-14.

[11] Anda, R. F., Felitti, V. J., Bremner, J. D., Walker, J. D., Whitfield, C., Perry, B. D., Dube, S. R., & Giles W. H. (2006). The enduring effects of abuse and related adverse experiences in childhood: A convergence of evidence from neurobiology and epidemiology. *European Archives of Psychiatry and Clinical Neuroscience, 256,* 174-86.

[12] Levine, P. & Phillips, P. (2012). *Freedom from Pain: Discover Your*

Body's Power to Overcome Physical Pain. Sounds True.

[13] Schubiner. *Unlearn Your Pain. Mind*Body*, 30.

[14] Dunbar, R., Baron, R., Frangou, A., Pearce, E., van Leeuwen, E., Stow, J., Partridge, G., MacDonald, I., Barra V and van Vugt, M.. (2012). Social laughter is correlated with an elevated pain threshold. *Proceedings of the Royal Society of Biological Sciences*, 279, 11161-1167.

[15] Harte, J. L., Eifert, G. H., & Smith, R. (1995). The effects of running and meditation on beta-endorphin, corticotrophin-releasing hormone and cortisol in plasma, and on mood. *Biological Psychology, 40(3)*, 251-65.

[16] Harte. (1995). The effects of running and meditation on beta-endorphin . . .

[17] Pert, C. (1999). *Molecules of Emotion*. New York: Simon and Schuster.

[18] Sprouse-Blum, A., Smith, G., Sugai, D., & Parsa D. (2010). Understanding endorphins and their importance in pain management. *Hawaii Medical Journal, 69*, 70-71.

[19] Sveinsdotir, V., Eriksen, H.R., & Reme, S.E. (2012) Assessing the role of cognitive behavioral therapy in the management of chronic nonspecific back pain. *Journal of Pain Research, 5*, 371-80.

[20] Brox, J. I., Sorensen, R., Friis, A. et Al. (2003). Randomized clinical trial of lumbar instrumented fusion and cognitive intervention and exercises in patients with chronic low-back pain and disc degeneration. *Spine, 28*(17), 1913–1921.

[21] Brox J. I., Reikeras, O., Nygaard, O., et al. (2006). Lumbar instrumented fusion compared with cognitive intervention and exercises in patients with chronic back pain after previous surgery for disc herniation: a prospective randomized controlled study. *Pain,* 122(1–2), 145–155.

[22] Brox, J. I., Nygaard, O. P., Holm, I., Keller, A., Ingebrigtsen, T., & Reikeras, O. (2010). Four-year follow-up of surgical versus non-surgical therapy for chronic low-back pain. *Ann Rheum Dis, 69*(9), 1643–1648.

[23] Keller, A., Brox, J. I., Gunderson, R., Holm, I., Friis, A., & Reikeras, O. (2004). Trunk muscle strength, cross-sectional area, and density in patients with chronic low-back pain randomized to lumbar fusion or cognitive intervention and exercises. *Spine, 29*(1):3–8.

[24] Froholdt, A., Holm, I., Keller, A., Gunderson, R. B., Reikeraas, O., & Brox, J. I. (2011), No difference in long-term trunk muscle strength, cross-sectional area, and density in patients with chronic low-back pain 7 to 11 years after lumbar fusion versus cognitive intervention and exercises. *The Spine Journal, 11*(8), 718–725.

[25] Fairbank, J., Frost, H., Wilson-MacDonald, J., Yu, L. M., Barker, K., & Collins, R. (2005). Randomised controlled trial to compare surgical stabilisation of the lumbar spine with an intensive rehabilitation programme for patients with chronic low-back pain: the MRC spine stabilisation trial. *BMJ, 330*(7502), 1233.

[26] Carroll, D. (1998). Relaxation for the relief of chronic pain: a systematic review. *Journal of Advanced Nursing, 27*, 476-487.

[27] NIH Technology Assessment Panel of Integration of Behavioral and Relaxation Approaches into the Treatment of Chronic Pain and Insomnia, Integration of behavioral and relaxation approaches into the treatment of chronic pain and insomnia. (1996). *JAMA, 276*(4), 313-8.

[28] Yucha, C. & Montgomery, C. (2008). *Evidence-Based Practice in Biofeedback, Association for Applied Psychophysiology and Biofeedback.*

[29] Flor, H. & Birbaumer, N. (1993). Comparison of the efficacy of electromyographic biofeedback, cognitive-behavioral therapy and conservative medical interventions in the treatment of chronic musculoskeletal pain. *Journal of Consulting and Clinical Psychology, 61*(4), 653-658.

[30] Corrado, P., Gottlieb, H., & Abdelhamid, M. H. (2003). The effect of biofeedback and relaxation training on anxiety and somatic complaints in chronic pain patients. *American Journal of Pain Management, 13*(4), 133-139.

[31] Humphreys, P. A., & Gevirtz, R. (2000). Treatment of recurrent abdominal pain: Components analysis of four treatment protocols. *Journal of Pediatric Gastroenterological Nutrition, 31*(1), 47-51.

[32] Vasudeva, S., Claggett, A. L., Tietjen, G. E., & McGrady, A. V. (2003). Biofeedback-assisted relaxation in migraine headache: Relationships to cerebral blood flow velocity in the middle cerebral artery. *Headache, 43*(3), 245-50.

[33] Rokicki, L. A., Holroyd, K. A., Brance, C. R., Lipchik, G.L., France, J. L., & Kvaal, S. A. (1997). Change mechanisms associated with

combined relaxation/EMG biofeedback training for chronic tension headache. *Applied Psychophysiology and Biofeedback, 22*(1), 21-41.

[34] Silberstein, S. D. (2000). Practice parameter: Evidence-based guidelines for migraine headaches (an evidence-based review): Report of the quality standards subcommittee of the American Academy of Neurology. *Neurology, 55*, 754-762.

[35] Hargrove, J. B., Bennett, R. M., Simons, D. G., Smith, S. J., Naqpal, S., Deering, D. E. (2010). Quantitative electroencephalographic abnormalties in fibromyalgia patients. *Clinical EEG and Neuroscience, 4*(3), 132-9.

[36] Stern, J., Jeanmonod, D., & Sarnthein, J. (2006). Persistent EEG overactivation in the cortical pain matrix of neurogenic pain patients. *Neuroimage, 31*(2), 721-31.

[37] Prichep, L .S., John, E. R., Howard, B., Merkin, H, & Hiesiger, E. M. (2001). Evaluation of the pain matrix using EEG source localization: a feasibility study. *Pain Medicine, 12*(8), 1241-8.

[38] Jensen, M. P., Sherlin, L. H., Gertz, K. J., Braden, A. L., Kupper, A. E., Gianas, A., Howe, J. D., & Hakimian, S. (2013) Brain EEG activity correlates of chronic pain in persons with spinal cord injury: clinical implications. *Spinal Cord, 51*(1), 55-8.

[39] Kayiram, S., Dursun, E., Dursun. N, Ermutlu, N, Karamursel S. (2010). Neurofeedback intervention in fibromyalgia syndrome; a randomized controlled rater blind clinical trial. *Applied Psychophysiology and Biofeedback, 35*(4), 293-302.

[40] Walker, J. (2011). QEEG-guided neurofeedback for recurrent migraine headaches. *Clinical EEG and Neuroscience, 42*(1), 59-61.

[41] Jensen, M. P., Gertz, K. J., Kupper, A. E., Braden, A. L., Howe, J. D., Kakimian, S., & Sherlin, L. H. (2013). Steps toward developing an EEG biofeedback treatment for chronic pain. *Applied Psychophysiology and Biofeedback, 38*(2), 101-8.

[42] Schubiner. Unlearn Your Pain. Mind*Body, 5.

[43] Schubinder. Unlearn Your Pain. Mind*Body, 44-48.

[44] Sarno, J. (2010). *Healing Back Pain.* New York: Grand Central Life & Style.

[45] Sarno J. (2001). *The Mind/Body Prescription* Grand Central Publishing.

[46]http://www.tmswiki.org/ppd/The_20/20_segment_on_John_Sarno_and_ TMS accessed on 8/4/13.

[47] Schubiner. *Unlearn Your Pain. Mind*Body*, 72-73

[48] Schubiner. *Unlearn Your Pain. Mind*Body*, 157.

[49] Schubiner. *Unlearn Your Pain. Mind*Body*, 15.

[50] Pennebaker, J. (1997). *Opening Up: the Healing Power of Expressing Emotions.* New York: The Guilford Press, 9-10.

[51] Pennebaker. *Opening Up.* Guilford, 7.

[52] Levine & Phillips. *Freedom from Pain.* Sounds True, 3.

[53] Schnurr, P. & Green, B. (2003). *Physical Health Consequences of Extreme Stress,* American Psychological Association, Washington, 3-10.

[54] Geissr, M. E., Rptj, R. S., Bachman, J. E., & Exkert, T. A. (1996). The relationship between symptoms of post-traumatic stress disorder and pain, affective disturbance and disability among patients with accident and non-accident related pain. *Pain, 66*(2-3), 207-214,

[55] Levine & Phillips. *Freedom from Pain.* Sounds True, 5-6.

[56] Shapiro, F. (1989) Eye Movement Desensitization: A new treatment for posttraumatic stress disorder. *Journal of Behavior Therapy & Experimental Psychiatry, 20*(3), 211-217.

[57] Van Rood, Y. & de Roos, C. (2009). EMDR in the treatment of medically unexplained symptoms: a systematic review. *Journal of EMDR Practice and Research, 3*(4), 248-63.

[58] Grant, M. (2012). *Pain Control with EMDR: Treatment Manual.* Mark Grant, 47.

[59] Grant. (2012). *Pain Control with EMDR*, 49.

[60] Grant. (2012). *Pain Control with EMDR*, 48.

[61] Grant. (2012). *Pain Control with EMDR*, 50

[62] Grant. (2012). *Pain Control with EMDR*, .51

[63] Grant. (2012). *Pain Control with EMDR*, 82-84.

[64] Schneider, J., Hofmann, A., Rost, C., & Shapiro, F. (2008). EMDR in the treatment of chronic phantom limb pain. *Pain Medicine, 9*, 76–82.

[65] Wilensky, M. (2006). Eye movement desensitization and reprocessing (EMDR) as a treatment for phantom limb pain. *J Brief Ther, 5*, 31–44.

[66] de Roos, C., Veenst,ra A. C., de Jongh, A., et al. (2010). Treatment of chronic phantom limb pain using a trauma-focused psychological approach. *Pain Res Manag, 15*, 55-71, 65–71.

[67] Marcus, S. V. (2008). Phase 1 of integrated EMDR: An abortive treatment for migraine headaches. *Journal of EMDR Practice Research, 2*, 15–25.

[68] Konuk, E., Epözdemir, H., Atçeken, S., Aydin YE., & Yurtsever, A. (2011). EMDR treatment of migraine. *Journal of EMDR Practice Research, 5*, 166–76.

[69] Grant, M., Threlfo C. (2002). EMDR in the treatment of chronic pain. *Journal of Clinical Psychology, 58*, 1505–20.

[70] Hassard, A. (1995). Investigation of eye movement desensitization in pain clinic patients. *Behav Cogn Psychother, 23*, 177–85.

[71] Allen, T. M. (2004*). Efficacy of EMDR and chronic pain management.* Chicago: Argosy University.

[72] Kavakcı, O., Semiz, M., Kaptanoglu, E., & Ozer, Z. (2012). EMDR treatment in fibromyalgia, a study of seven cases. *Anatolian Journal of Psychiatry, 13*, 75–81.

[73] Friedberg, F. (2004). Eye movement desensitization in fibromyalgia: A pilot study. *Complementary Therapy in Nursing Midwifery, 10*, 245–9.

[74] Mazzola, A., Calcagno, M. L., Goicochea, M. T., et al. (2009). EMDR in the treatment of chronic pain. *Journal of EMDR Practice Research, 3*, 66–79.

[75] Tesarz, J., Leisner, S., Gerhardt, A., Janke, S., Seidler, G. H., Eich, W., & Hartmann, M. (2014). Effects of eye movement desensitization and reprocessing (EMDR) treatment in chronic pain patients: a systematic review. *Pain Medicine, 15*(2), 247-63.

[76] Tesrz, J., Gerhardt, A., Leisner, S., Janke, S., Hartmann, M., Seidler, G., & Eich, W. (2013). Effects of eye movement desensitization and reprocessing (EMDR) o. CAM and energy psychology techniques remediate PTSD symptoms in veterans and spouses n non-specific chronic back pain: a randomized controlled trial with additional exploration of the underlying mechanisms. *BMC Musculoskeletal*

Disorders, 14, 256.

[77] Association for Comprehensive Energy Psychology. The state of energy psychology research. http://www.energypsych.org/?Research_Landing

[78] Association for Comprehensive Energy Psychology. What is Energy Psychology? http://www.energypsych.org/?AboutEPv2

[79] Lane, J. (2009). The neurochemistry of counterconditioning: acupressure desensitization in psychotherapy. *Energy Psychology: Theory, Research and Treatment, 1,* 31-44.

[80] Church, D., & Brooks, A. J. (2014). *Explore: The Journal of Science and Healing, 10*(1), 24-33.

[81] Bougea, A. M., Spandideas, N., Alexopoulos, E. C., Thomaides, T., Chrousos, G. P., & Darviri, C. (2013). Effect of the Emotional Freedom Technique on Perceived Stress, Quality of Life, and Cortisol Salivary Levels in Tension-Type Headache Sufferers: A Randomized Controlled Trial. *EXPLORE: The Journal of Science and Healing, 9*(2), 91-99.

[82] Brattberg, G. (20008). Self-administered EFT (Emotional Freedom *Techniques*) in individuals with fibromyalgia: a randomized trial. *Integrative Medicine: A Clinician's Journal,* 30-35.

[83] Church, D. & Brooks, A. (2010). The Effect of a Brief EFT (Emotional Freedom Techniques) Self-Intervention on Anxiety, Depression, Pain and Cravings in Healthcare Workers. *Integrative Medicine: A Clinician's Journal,* 40-44.

[84] Video. www.youtube.com/user/CareyMannTV.

[85] Ortner, N. (2015). *The Tapping Solution for Pain Relief: A Step-by-Step Guide to Reducing and Eliminating Chronic Pain.* New York: Hay House.

[86] Barber J. (1996)A brief introduction to hypnotic analgesia, in Barber J, *Hypnosis and Suggestion in the Treatment of Pain: A Clinical Guide,* W.W. Norton & Company, New York,5.

[87] Barber. (1996). A brief introduction to hynpotic analgesia, 6.

[88] Barber. (1996). A brief introduction to hynpotic analgesia, 25-26.

[89] Barber. (1996). A brief introduction to hynpotic analgesia, 10.

[90] Barber. (1996). A brief introduction to hynpotic analgesia, 14-16.

[91] Fass, S, (2008). Hypnosis for Pain Management in Weintraub M, Mamtani R ad Micozzi M, *Complementary and Integrative Medicine in Pain Management*, Springer Publishing Company, New York, 30-31.

[92] Fass. (2008). Hypnosis for Pain Management, 31.

[93] Montgomery, G. H, DuHamel, K. N., & Redd, W. H. (2000). A meta-analysis of hypnotically induced analgesia: how effective is hypnosis? *International Journal of Clinical and Experimental Hypnosis, 48*(2), 138-153.

[94] Jensen, M. & Patterson, D. (2006). Hypnotic treatment of chronic pain. *Journal of Behavioral Medicine, 29*, 95-124.

[95] Fass. (2008). Hypnosis for Pain Management, 38-39.

[96] Substance Abuse and Mental Health Services Administration Report to Congress on the Nation's Substance Abuse and Mental Health Workforce Issues. (2013.)

Chp. 6: Manipulative and Body-Based Practices (87–109)

[1] Plamondon, R. (1995). Summary of 1994 ACA annual statistical study. *Journal of the American Chiropractic Association, 32*(1), 57-63.

[2] Coulter, I., (1998). Efficacy and risks of chiropractic manipulation: What does the evidence suggest? *Integrative Medicine, 1*(2), 61-66.

[3] Cherkin, D. C.., Mootz, R. D., (eds.) (1997). Chiropractic in the United States: training, practice and research. Rockville, Maryland: Agency for Health Care Policy and Research, Public Health Service, US Department of Health and Human Services. AHCPR Publication No. 98-N002.

[4] Bigos, S., et al. (1994). *Acute Lower Back Pain in Adults, Clinical Practice Guideline Quick Reference Guide Number 14* Rockville, MD: US Department of Health and Human Services, Public Health Service, Agency for Health Care Policy and Research.

[5] Rosen, M. (1994) *Back Pain: Report of a Clinical Standards Advisory Group Committee on Back Pain*, London, England: HMSO.

[6] Commission on Alternative Medicine. (1987) *Social Departementete: Legitimization for vissa kiropraktorer*, 12, 13-16.

[7] Danish Institute for Health Technology Assessment 1999.

[8] Thompson, C. J. (1986). *Second Report, Medicare Benefits Review*

Committee. Canberra, Australia: Commonwealth Government Printer.

[9] Hassellberg, P. D. (1979). *Chiropractic in New Zealand: Report of a Commission of Inquiry.* Wellington, New Zealand, Government Printer.

[10] Jonas, W. (2000). Forward to Chapman-Smith, D., *The Chiropractic Profession,* NMIC Group, Inc.

[11] Personal interview.

[12] Jonas, W. (2000). Forward to Chapman-Smith, 15.

[13] Jonas, W. (2000). Forward to Chapman-Smith, 17.

[14] Personal interview.

[15] http://www.chiro.org/Wilk/

[16] Chapman-Smith, David. (2000). *The Chiropractic Profession.* NMIC Group, Inc, 1.

[17] *Occupational Outlook Handbook, January 8, 2014,* Bureau of Labor Statistics, US Department of Labor http://www.bls.gov/ooh/healthcare/chiropractors.htm

[18] Foreman, S. & Stahl, M. (2010) The attrition rate of licensed chiropractors in California: an exploratory ecological investigation of time-trend data. Chiropractic & Osteopathy, 18(24).

[19] Coulter ID, Shekelle PG. (1997) Supply, Distribution and Utilization of Chiropractors in the United States. In *Chiropractic in the United States: Training, Practice and Research* (AHCPR Publication no. 98-N002), Cherkin, D. C. & Mootz, R. (eds.), (!997), Rockville, MD: Agency for Health Care Policy and Research, Public Health Service, US Department of Health and Human Services.

[20] Eisenberg, D. M, Davis, R. B, & Ettner, S. L. et al. (1998). Trends in alternative medicine use in the United States, 1990-1997: results of a followup national survey. *JAMA, 280*(18), 1569-1575.

[21] Cooper, R. & McKee, H. (2003). Chiropractic in the United States: Trends and Issues. *The Milbank Quarterly, 81*(1), 120.

[22] Barnes, P. M, Powell-Griner, E., McFann, K., Nahin, R. L. (2004). Complementary and alternative medicine use among adults: United States. *Adv Data, 27*(343), 1-19.

[23] Bachinger, E., Bauer, R., Ritter, H. Gesundheitbericht fur Wien 1998.

Stadt Wien. 1999.

[24] Haertel, U. & Volger E. (2004). Use and acceptance of classical natural and alternative medicine in Germany—findings of a representative population-based survey. *Forsch Komplementarmed Klass Naturheilkd, 11*(6), 327-334.

[25] American Physical Therapy Association. Role of a physical therapist. ttp://www.apta.org/PTCareers/RoleofaPT/ accessed on 11/22/14.

[26] http://www.webmd.com/pain-management/tc/physical-therapy-topic-overview accessed on 11/23/14.

[27] http://www.webmd.com/hw-popup/manual-therapy accessed on 11/23/14.

[28] http://www.webmd.com/pain-management/tc/physical-therapy-topic-overview accessed on 11/23/14.

[29] http://education-portal.com/physical_therapy_certification.html accessed on 11/23/15.

[30] http://en.wikipedia.org/wiki/Physical_therapy accessed on 11/23/14.

[31] Watson, P. (2007). Soft tissue pain and physical therapy. *Anaesthesia and Intensive Care Medicine, 9*(1), 27-28.

[32] Stanos S., Muellner, P. M., & Harden, R. M. (2004). The physiatric approach to low-back pain. *Seminars in Pain Medicine, 2,* 186-196.

[33] Bokarius, A. & Bokarius, V. (2010). Evidence-based review of manual therapy efficacy in treatment of chronic musculoskeletal pain. *Pain Practice, 10*(5), 451-458.

[34] Pignolet, J. (2013, February 3). Physical therapy booms with aging, active seniors. *The Spokesman Review.*

[35] Fritz, J., Hunter, S., Tracy, D., & Brennan, G. (2011). Utilization and clinical outcomes of outpatient physical therapy for Medicare beneficiaries with musculoskeletal conditions. *Physical Therapy, 91,* 330-345.

[36] Information based on numerous interviews with physical therapists.

[37] US Bureau of Labor Statistics. http://www.bls.gov/ooh/healthcare/physical-therapists.htm#tab-6 on December 28, 2014.

[38] Personal interview.

[39] Personal interview.

[40] Personal interview.

[41] Personal interview.

[42] Madore, A. & Kahn, J. R. (2008). Therapeutic Massage and Bodywork in Integrative Pain Management in *Contemporary Pain Medicine: Integrative Pain Medicine: The Science and Practice of Complementary and Alternative Medicine in Pain Management.* Audette, J. F. & Bailey, A. (eds.). Totowa, NJ: Humana Press, 363.

[43] IBIS World Industry Report OD6028 Massage Services, January 2014.

[44] American Massage Therapy Association Industry Fact Sheet. http://www.amtamassage.org/infocenter/economic_industry-factsheet.html?src=navdropdown#Who on 2/15/15

[45] American Massage Therapy Association Industry Fact Sheet.

[46] Madore, A. & Kahn, J. R. (2008). Therapeutic Massage and Bodywork in Integrative Pain Management, 355.

[47] Cherkin, D. C, Eisenberg, D., Sherman, K. J., Barlow, W., Kaptchuk, T. J., Street, J., & Deyo, R. A. (2001). Randomized trial comparing traditional Chinese medical acupuncture, therapeutic massage, and self-care education for chronic low-back pain. *Archives of Internal Medicine, 161*(8), 1081-8.

[48] Sherman, K. J., Cherkin, D. C., Hawkes, R. J. et al. (2006). Randomized trial of therapeutic massage versus self-care book for chronic neck pain. Presented at North American Research Conference on Complementary and Integrative Medicine, Edmonton.

[49] Perlman. A., Mojica, E., Williams, A_L et al. Massage therapy for osteoarthritis of the knee: results of randomized controlled trial. Presentation at North American Research Conference on Complementary and Integrative Medicine, Edmonton, Mary 23-26, 2006.

[50] Furlan, A. D., Imamura, M., Dryden, T., & Irvin, E. (2008). Massage for low-back pain. *Cochrane Database of Systematic Reviews* (4). Art. No.: CD001929.

[51] Cherkin, D. C., Sherman, I., Kahn, K., Wellman, R., Cook, A., Johnson, E., Erro, J., Delaney, K., Deyo, R. (2011). A comparison of the effects of 2 types of massage and usual care on chronic low-back pain: a randomized controlled trial. *Annals of Internal Medicine,*

155(1), 1-9.

[52] Majchrzycki, M., Kocur, P., & Kotwiki, T. (2014). Deep Tissue Massage and nonsteroidal anti-inflammatory drugs for low-back pain: a prospective randomized trial. *The Scientific World Journal*, 1-7.

[53] Yuan, S. L., Matsutani, L. A, & Marques, A. P. (2014). Effectiveness of different styles of massage therapy in fibromyalgia: A systematic review and meta-analysis. *Manual Therapy*. E-published ahead of print on Oct 5, 2014.

[54] Li, Y., Wang, F., Feng, C., Yang, X., & Sun, Y. (2014). Massage therapy for fibromyalgia: a systematic review and meta-analysis of randomized controlled trials. *PLoS One*, 9(2):e89304.

[55] Davidson, A., personal communication.

[56] Jacobson, E. (2011). Structural integration, an alternative method of manual therapy and sensorimotor education. *The Journal of Alternative and Complementary Medicine*, 17(10), 891-899.

[57] Jacobson. (2011). Structural integration.

[58] Jacobson. (2011). Structural integration.

[59] Deutsch, J., Derr, L. L., Judd, P., & Reuven, B. (2000). Treatment of chronic pain through the use of Structural Integration (Rolfing). *Orthopedic and Physical Therapy Clinics of North America, 9*, 411–427.

[60] James, H., Castaneda, L., Miller, M. E., & Findley, T. (2009). Rolfing structural integration treatment of cervical spine dysfunction. *Journal of Bodywork and Movement Therapy, 13*, 229–238.

[61] Personal interview

[62] http://www.nmtcenters.com/about-neuromuscular-therapy.php accessed on 3/8/15.

[63] http://www.nmtcenters.com/about-neuromuscular-therapy.php accessed on 3/8/15.

Chp. 7: Nutritional Interventions (pp. 111–147)

[1] Sulindro-Ma, M., Ivy, C., & Isenhart, A. (2008). Nutrition and Supplements for Pain Management, in *Integrative Pain Medicine: The Science and Practice of Complementary and Alternative Medicine in Pain Management*. Audette, J. F. & Bailey, A. Totowa, NJ: Humana Press, 418.

[2] Sulindo-Ma & Isenhart. (2008). Nutrition and Supplements for Pain Management.

[3] Meleger, A. L., Froude, C. K., & Walker, J. 3rd. (2014). Nutrition and eating behavior in patients with chronic pain receiving long-term opioid therapy. *PM&R*, *6*(1), 7-12.

[4] http://www.who.int/mediacentre/news/notes/2014/consultation-sugar-guideline/en/ accessed on 5/31/14.

[5] Sulindo-Ma & Isenhart. (2008). Nutrition and Supplements for Pain Management, 419.

[6] Sulindo-Ma & Isenhart. (2008). Nutrition and Supplements for Pain Management.

[7] http://articles.mercola.com/sites/articles/archive/2011/11/11/everything-you-need-to-know-about-fatty-acids.aspx accessed on 9/13/14.

[8] Sulindo-Ma & Isenhart. (2008). Nutrition and Supplements for Pain Management, 420.

[9] Maroon, J. C. & Bost, J. W. (2006). Omega-3 fatty acids (fish oil)as an inti-inflammatory: an alternative to nonsteroidal anti-inflammatory drugs for discogenic pain. *Surgical Neurology*, *65*(4), 326-31.

[10] Ramsden, C. E., Faurot, K. R., Zamora, D., Suchindran, C. M., Macintosh, B. A., Gaylord, S. . . . Mann, J. D. (2013). Targeted alteration of dietary n-3 and n-6 fatty acids for the treatment of chronic headaches. *Pain*, *154*(11), 2441-51.

[11] Lee, Y. H., Bae, S. C., & Song, G. G. (2012). Omega-3 polyundaturated fatty acids and the treatment of rheumatoid arthritis: a meta-analysis. *Archives of Medical Research*, *43*(5), 356-62.

[12] Uchiyama, K., Nakamura, M., Odahara, S., Koido, S., Katahira, K., Shiraishi, H., Ohkusa, T., Fujise, K., &Tajiri, H. (2010). N-3 polyunsaturated fatty acid diet therapy for patients with inflammatory bowel disease. *Inflammatory Bowel Disease*, *16*(10), 1696-707.

[13] Cuda, A. (2008). Fish oil replaces NSAIDS. *Massage Magazine*, 108.

[14] http://articles.mercola.com/sites/articles/archive/2014/02/17/vitamin-d-supplements.aspx accessed on 5/31/14.

[15] Birkner, K. (2010). Chronic Pain and Vitamin D. *HER-92*. *Pain and Stress Publications*.

[16] Birkner. (2010). Chronic Pain and Vitamin D.

[17] Sulindo-Ma & Isenhart. (2008). Nutrition and Supplements for Pain Management, 421.

[18] Vasquez, A. (2004). Vitamin D supplementation in the treatment of musculoskeletal pain. *The Original Internist*, 07.

[19] Trang, H. M, Cole, D. E, Rubin, L. A, Pierratos, A., Siu, S., Vieth, R. (1998). Evidence that vitamin D3 increases serum 25-hydroxyvitamin D more efficiently than does vitamin D2. *American Journal of Clinical Nutrition, 68*, 854-8.

[20] Amas, L. A., Hollis, B. W., & Heaney, R. P. (2004). Vitamin D2 is much less effective than Vitamin D3 in humans. *Journal of Clinical Endocrimology Metabolism, 89*, 5387-91.

[21] People with undetermined muscle/bone pain tend to be severely vitamin D deficient. Public release: December 9, 2003, Minneapolis, St. Paul. Contact: ashleyb@umn.edu, University of Minnesota.

[22] Plotnikoff, G. A. & Quigley, J. M. (2003). Prevalence of severe hypovitaminosis D in pateints with persistent, nonspecific musculoskeletal pain. *Mayo Clin Proc, 78*, 1463-1470.

[23] Birkner. (2010). Chronic Pain and Vitamin D.

[24] Autler, P., Boniol, M., Pizot, C., & Mullie, P. (2014). Vitamin D status and ill health: a systematic review. *The Lancet Diabetes & Endocrinology, 2*(1):76-89.

[25] Gloth, F. M. 3rd, Lindsay, J. M., Zelesnick, L. B., & Greenough, W. B. 3rd. (1991) Can vitamin D deficiency produce an unusual pain syndrome? *Archives of Internal Medicine, 151*(8), 1662-4.

[26] Schreuder, F., Bernsen, R. M., vn der Wouden, J. C. (2012). Vitamin D supplementation for nonspecific musculoskeletal pain in non-Western immigrants: a randomized controlled trial. *Annals of Family Medicine, 10*(6):547-55.

[27] Sanghi, D., Mishra, A., Sharma, A. C., Singh, A., Natu, S. M., Agarwal, S., & Srivastava, R. N. (2013). Does Vitamin D improve osteoarthritis of the knee: a randomized controlled pilot trial. *Clinical Orthopedics and Related Research*, (11), 3556-62.

[28] Huaang, W., Shah, S., Long, Q., Crankshaw, A. K., & Tangpricha, V. (2013). *The Clinical Journal of Pain*, (4), 341-7.

[29] Osunkwo, I., Ziegler, T. R., McCracken, C., Cherry, K., Osunkwo, C. E.,

Ofori-Acquah, S. F., Ghosh, S., Ogungobode, A., Eckman, J. R., Dampier, C., & Tangprich, V. (2012) *British Jouranl of Haematology, 159*(2), 211-5.

[30] Jancin, B. (2013). Vitamin D promising in women with diabetic pain. *Internal Medicine News, 46*(13), 35.

[31] Kragstrup, T. W. (2011). Vitamin D supplementation for patients with chronic pain. *Scandinavian Journal of Primary Health Care*, (29), 4-5.

[32] http://articles.mercola.com/sites/articles/archive/2014/02/17/vitamin-d-supplements.aspx accessed on 5/31/14.

[33] O'Connor, A. (2014). Vitamin D screening not backed by expert panel *New York Times*.

[34] http://articles.mercola.com/sites/articles/archive/2014/02/17/vitamin-d-supplements.aspx

[35] Yousef, A. & Al-deeb, E. (2013). A double-blinded randomised controlled study of the value of sequential intravenous and oral magnesium therapy in patients with chronic low-back pain with a neuropathic component. *Anaesthesia*, (68), 260-266.

[35] Collins, S., Zuumond, W., de Lange, J., van Hilten, B., & Perez, R. (2009). Intravenous Magnesium for Complex Regional Pain Syndrome Type 1 (CRPS1) Patients: A Pilot Study. *Pain Medicine, 10*(5), 930-40.

[36] Bagis, S., Karabiber, M., As, I., Tamer, L., Erdogan, C., & Atalay A. (2013). Is magnesium citrate treatment effective on pain, clinical parameters and functional status in patients with fibromyalgia? *Rheumatology International, 33*(1), 167-72.

[37] De Francesschi, L., Bachir, D., Galacteros, F., Tchernia, G., Cynober, T., Neuberg, D., Beuzard, Y., & Brugnara. (2000). Oral magnesium pidolate: effects of long term administration in patients with sickle cell disease. *British Journal of Haematology*, (108), 284-289.

[38] Personal interview.

[39] Emord, J. (2010). *Global Censorship of Health Information*, Washington, DC: Sentinel Press, 1.

[40] Emord. (2010). *Global Censorship of Health Information*, 2.

[41] Emord. (2010). *Global Censorship of Health Information*, 30-31.

[42] Emord. (2010). *Global Censorship of Health Information*, 10.

[43] Emord. (2010). *Global Censorship of Health Information*, 16.

[44] Emord. (2010). *Global Censorship of Health Information*, 33.

[45] Personal interview.

[46] Alliance for Natural Health. The FDA's New Sneak Attack on Supplements (2011, July 5). http://www.anh-usa.org/fda-new-sneak-attack-on-supplements/.

[47] Minton, M. (2011, July 28). The coming war on vitamins: New FDA rules would diminish nutrient choices. *Washington Times*.

[48] Minton, M. (2011). *The Coming War on Vitamins*.

[49] http://www.anh-usa.org/dietary-supplement-labeling-act-a-huge-smokescreen/ accessed on 11/28/11.

[50] http://www.crnusa.org/CRNPR10_CRNquestionsaccuracyofherbalstudy020110.html accessed on 12/4/11.

[51] http://www.medalerts.org/vaersdb/findfield.php?TABLE=ON&GROUP1=AGE&ONSET_YEAR_LOW=2008&ONSET_YEAR_HIGH=2008

[52] http://www.fda.gov/Drugs/GuidanceComplianceRegulatoryInformation/Surveillance/AdverseDrugEffects/ucm070434.htm accessed on 12/4/11.

[53] http://www.anh-usa.org/durbin-and-waxman-strike-again/ accessed on 11/28/11.

[54] http://www.anh-usa.org/durbin-and-waxman-strike-again/ accessed on 11/28/11.

[55] Dietary supplements cause 600 "adverse events." (2008). *USA Today*.

[56] ECJ Ruling Secures Future for Vitamins and Minerals, ANH Press Release. (2005).

[57] UK Regulatory Impact Assessment on UK Regulations implementing FSD

[58] www.anh-europe.org

[59] www.anh-europe.org

[60] Opinion of Advocate General Geelhoed, Joined cases C-154/04 and C-155/04, April 5, 2005.

[61] *IVR Encyclopedia of Jurisprudence*, Legal Theory and Philosophy of

Law

[62]Opinion of Advocate General Geelhoed, Joined cases C-154/04 and C-155/04, April 5, 2005.

[63] ECJ Ruling Secures Future for Vitamins and Minerals, ANH Press Release. (2005).

[64] ECJ Ruling Secures Future for Vitamins and Minerals. (2005).

[65] http://www.celiaccentral.org/newlydiagnosed/What-is-Celiac-Disease/1103/ accessed on 9/13/14.

[66] http://www.celiaccentral.org/newlydiagnosed/Celiac-Symptoms/32/ accessed on 9/13/14.

[67] http://www.celiaccentral.org/non-celiac-gluten-sensitivity/introduction-and-definitions/

[68] Stump, J. (2003). Acupuncture Management of Celiac Disease. *Medical Acupuncture, 14*(3), 38-40.

[69] Magnuson, B. A., Burdock, G. A., Doull, J., Kroes, R. M., Marsh, G. M., Pariza, M. W. . . . Williams, G. M. (2007). Aspartame: a safety evaluation based on current use levels, regulations, and toxicological and epidemiological studies. *Critical Reviews in Toxicology, 37*(8), 629-727.

[70] Magnuson et al. (2007). Aspartame.

[71] Aspartame Toxicity Information Center. http://www.HolisticMed.com/aspartame/.

[72] Yang, Q. (2010). Gain weight by "going diet?" Artificial sweeteners and the neurobiology of sugar cravings. *Yale Journal of Biology and Medicine, 83*(2), 101-108.

[73] Marcus, N., MD. (2012). *End Back Pain Forever: A Groundbreaking Approach to Eliminate Your Suffering.* Atria Books, 199.

Chp. 8: Herbal Treatments (pp. 149–159)

[1] Low Dog, T. (2009).Botanicals in the management of pain. In *Contemporary Pain Medicine: Integrative Pain Medicine: The Science and Practice of Complementary and Alternative Medicine in Pain Management.* Audette, J. F. & Bailey, A. (eds.) Totowa, NJ: Humana Press, 447.

[2] Low Dog. (2009). Botanicals in the management of pain, 448

[3] Low Dog. (2009). Botanicals in the management of pain, 448.

[4] Chamberland, G. (2011). *The Use of Herbal Remedies in the Treatment of Pain: Natural Pain Management & Herbal Remedies as Complementary Medicine.* Curaphyte Technologies.

[5] Chamberland. (2011). *The Use of Herbal Remedies.*

[6] Thomson Healthcare. (2007). *PDR for Herbal Medicines, 4th Edition.* Thompson Reuters.

[7] Hamidpour, R., Hamidpour, S., & Shahlari, M. (2013). Frankincense (乳香 Rǔ Xiāng; *Boswellia*Species): From the Selection of Traditional Applications to the Novel Phytotherapy for the Prevention and Treatment of Serious Diseases. *Journal of Traditional and Complementary Medicine, 3*(4), 221-226.

[8] Blanco, J. (2014). Report: Boswellia new studies show effective pain relief. *Life Extension Magazine* http://www.lifeextension.com//Magazine/2014/12/Boswellia-New-Studies-Show-Effective-Pain-Relief/Page-01 on July 20, 2015.

[9] Birkner, K. M. (2006). *Boswellia, The Pain Herb.* San Antonio, TX: Pain and Stress Publications.

[10] Kimmatkar, N., Thawani, V., Hingorani, L., & Khiyani, R. (2003). Efficacy and tolerability of Boswellia serrata extract in treatment of osteoarthritis of knee—a randomized double-blind placebo controlled trial. *Phytomedicine, 10*(1), 3-7.

[11] Sengupta, K., Alluri, K. V., Satish, A. R., et al. (2008). A double-blind, randomized placebo controlled study of the efficacy and safety of 5-Loxin for treatment of osteoarthritis of the knee. *Arthritis Res Ther*, 10(4), R85.

[12] Gupta, I., Parihar, A., Malhotra, P., et al. (1997). Effects of Boswellia serrata gum resin in patients with ulcerative colitis. *European Journal of Medical Research, 2*(1), 37-43

[13] Gupta, I., Parihar, A., Malhotra, P., et al. (2001). Effects of gum resin of Boswellia serrata in patients with chronic colitis. *Planta Med*, 67(5), 391-5.

[14] Birkner. (2010). Chronic Pain and Vitamin D.

[15] Platt, C. (2008). Preventing migraine pain with butterbur. *Life Extension Magazine*. http://www.lifeextension.com/magazine/2008/8/preventing-

migraine-pain-with-butterbur/page-01

[16] Holland, S., Silberstein, S. D., Freitag, F., Dodick, D. W., Argoff, C., & Ashman, E. (2012). Evidence-based guideline update: NSAIDS and other complementary treatments for episodic migraine prevention in adults. *Neurology, 78*:1346-53

[17] Grossmann, M. & Schmidramsl, H. (2000). An extract of Petasites hybridus is effective in the prophylaxis of migraine. *International Journal of Clinical Pharmacology and Therapeutics,* 38(9), 430-5.

[18] Lipton, R. B., Gobel, H., Einhaupl, K. M., Wilks, K., & Mauskop, A. (2004). Petasites hybridus root (butterbur) is an effective preventive treatment for migraine. *Neurology, 63*(12). 2240-4.

[19] Holland et al. (2012). Evidence-based guideline update.

[20] Foster, S. (2006). *Herbs for your health.* Loveland, CO: Interweave Press.

[21] Piscoya, J., Rodriguez, Z., Bustamante, S. A., Okuhama, N. N., Miller, M. J., & Sandoval, M. (2001). Efficacy and safety of freeze-dried cat's claw in osteoarthritis of the knee: mechanisms of action of the species Uncaria guianensis. *Inflammation Research* 2001, 50, 442–448.

[22] Mehta, K., Gala, J., Bhasale, S., Naik, S., Modak, M., Thakur, H., Deo, N., & Miller, M. (2007). Comparison of glucosamine sulfate and a polyherbal supplement for the relief of osteoarthritis of the knee: a randomized controlled trial. *BMC Complementary and Alternative Medicine,* 7(34).

[23] Mur, E., Hartig, F., Eibl, G., & Schirmer, M. (2002). Randomized double-blind trial of an extract from the pentacyclic alkaloid-chemotype of uncaria tomentosa for the treatment of rheumatoid arthritis. *Journal of Rheumatology,* (4), 678-81.

[24] Holland et al. (2012). Evidence-based guideline update.

[25] Pfaffenrath, V., Diener, H. C., Fischer, M., Friede, M., & Henneicke-von Zepelin, H. H. (2002). The efficacy and safety of Tanacetum parthenium (feverfew) in migraine prophylaxis–a double-blind, multicentre, randomized placebo-controlled dose-response study. *Cephalalgia,* 22. 523–532.

[26] Chamberland. (2011). *The Use of Herbal Remedies.*

[27] Akhtar, N. & Haqqi, T. M. (2012). Current nutraceuticals in the

management of osteoarthritis: a review. *Therapeutic Advances In Musculoskeletal Disease, 4*(3), 181-207.

[28] Bartels, E. M., Folmer, N. V., Bliddal, H., Altman, R. D., Juhl, C., Tarp, S., Zhang, W., & Christensen, R. (2015). Efficacy and safety of ginger in osteoarthritis patients: a meta-analysis of randomized placebo-controlled trials. *Osteoarthristis Cartilage*, (1), 12-21.

[29] Lakhan, S., Ford, C., & Tepper, D. (2015)> Zingiberaceae extracts for pain: a systematic review and meta-analysis. *Nutrition Journal*, 14:50.

[30] Akhtar & Haqqi. (2012). Current nutraceuticals in the management of osteoarthritis.

[31] Akhtar & Haqqi. (2012). Current nutraceuticals in the management of osteoarthritis.

[32] Aggarwal, B. B., Sudaram, C., Malani, N., & Ichikawa, H. (2007). Curcumin: the Indian solid gold. *Advances in Experimental Medicine and Biology*, 595, 1-75.

[33] Aggarwal et al. (2007). Curcumin.

[34] Chandran, B., Goel ,A. (2012). A randomized pilot study to assess the efficacy and safety of curcumin in patients with active rheumatoid arthritis. *Phytotherapy Research, 26*, 1719-25.

[35] Kuptniratsaikul, V., Dajpratham, P., Taechaarpornkul, W., Buntragulpoontawee, M., Lukkanapichonchut, P., Chootip, C., Saengsuwan, J., Tantayakom, K., & Laongpech, S. (2014). Efficacy and safety of Curcuma domestica extracts compared with ibuprofen in patients with knee osteoarthritis: a multicenter study. *Clinical Interventions in Aging, 9*, 451-8.

[36] Sharma, S., Chopra, K., & Kulkarni, S. K. (2007). Effect of insulin and its combination with resveratrol or curcumin in attenuation of diabetic neuropathic pain: participation of nitric oxide and TNF-alpha. *Phytotherapy Research, 21*, 278-83.

[37] Agarwal, K. A., Tripathi, C.D., Agarwal, B. B., & Saluja, S. (2011). Efficacy of turmeric (curcumin) in pain and postoperative fatigue after laparoscopic cholecystectomy: a double-blind, randomized placebo-controlled study. *Surgical Endoscopy, 25*, 3805-10.

[38] Vangsness, C. T., Spiker, W., & Erickson, J. (2009). A review of evidence-based medicine for glucosamine and chondroitin sulfate use in knee osteoarthritis. *Arthroscopy: The Journal of*

Arthroscopic and Related Surgery, 25(1), 86-94.

[39] Kolata, G. (2006, Febraury 6). Supplements fail to stop arthritis pain, study said. New York Times.

[40] Ibibucsi, L. & Poór, G. (1998). Efficacy and tolerability of oral chondroitin sulfate as a symptomatic slow-acting drug for osteoarthritis (SYSADOA) in the treatment of knee osteoarthritis. *Osteoarthritis Cartilage, 6*, 31-36 (suppl A).d.

[41] Conrozier, T. (1998). Anti-arthrosis treatments: Efficacy and tolerance of chondroitin sulfates (CS 4&6). *Presse Med, 27*, 1862-1865 (in French).

[42] Clegg, D., Reda, D. J., Harris, C. L., et al. (2006). Glucosamine, chondroitin sulfate, and the two in combination for painful knee osteoarthritis. *New England Journal of Medicine, 354*, 795-808

[43] Kolata. (2006). Supplements fail to stop arthritis pain.

[44] Walsh, N. (2015, January 21). Glucosamine and chondroitin: The OA evidence adds up—The supplements were as effective as Celebrex for knee pain. *Medpage Today*. http://ard.bmj.com/content/early/2015/01/14/annrheumdis-2014-on 8/7/15.

[45] Clegg. (2006). Glucosamine, chondroitin sulfate . . .

[46] Walsh. (2015). Glucosamine and chondroitin.

[47] Hochberg, M., Martel-Pelletier, J., Monfort, J., Moller, I., Castillo, J. R., Arden, N. . . . Pelletier, J. (2014). Combined chondroitin sulfate and glucosamine for painful knee osteoarthritis: a multicentre, randomised, double-blind, non-inferiority trial versus celecoxib. *Annals of the Rheumatic Diseases* http://ard.bmj.com/content/early/2015/01/14/annrheumdis-2014-206792.long

[48] Tant, L., Gillard, B., & Appelboom, T. (2005). Open-label, randomized controlled pilot study of the effects of a glucosamine complex on low-back pain. *Current Therapeutic Research, 66*(6), 511-21.

[49] Vangsness et al. (2009). A review of evidence-based medicine for glucosamine and chondroitin sulfate . . .

Chp. 9: Exercise (pp. 161–169)

[1] Marcus. (2012). *End Back Pain Forever*, 29.

[2] Marcus. (2012). *End Back Pain Forever*, 64.

[3] Marcus. (2012). *End Back Pain Forever*, 59.

[4] Marcus. (2012). *End Back Pain Forever*, 60-1.

[5] Marcus. (2012). *End Back Pain Forever*, 62-63.

[6] Marcus. (2012). *End Back Pain Forever*, 143.

[7] Marcus. (2012). *End Back Pain Forever*, 36.

[8] The Tampa Scale for Kinesiophobia assesses how much fear of injury is causing functional problems. https://www.tac.vic.gov.au/files-to-move/media/upload/tampa_scale_kinesiophobia.pdf. Higher scores mean that fear is interfering with recovery.

[9] http://www.bonnieprudden.com/blogs/where-are-my-muscle-weaknesses-%E2%80%93-and-what-do-i-do-about-them accessed on 10/14/14.

[10] Marcus. (2012). *End Back Pain Forever*, 36.

[11] Deyo, R.A. (2001). Weinstein J. Low-back pain. *New England Journal of Medicine, 344*(5), 363-370.

[12] Marcus. (2012). *End Back Pain Forever*, 56.

[13] Marcus. (2012). *End Back Pain Forever*, 4.

[14] Marcus. (2012). *End Back Pain Forever*, 35.

[15] Marcus. (2012). *End Back Pain Forever*, 94.

[16] Marcus. (2012). *End Back Pain Forever*, 95.

[17] Kraus, H., Nagler., & Melleby, A. (1983). Evaluation of an exercise program for back pain. *American Family Physician, 28*(3), 153-8.

[18] Marcus. (2012). *End Back Pain Forever*, 95.

[19] Marcus. (2012). *End Back Pain Forever*, 84.

[20] Hayden, J.A., van Tulder, M. W., & Tomlinson, G. Systematic review: strategies for using exercise therapy to improve outcomes in chronic low-back pain.

[21] O'Riordan, C, Cifford, A., Van De Ben, P., & Nelson, J. (2014). Chronic neck pain and exercise interventions: frequency, intensity, time and type principle. *Archives of Physical Medicine and Rehabilitation, 95*(4), 770-83.

[22] Bertozzi, L., Gardenghi, I., Turoni, F., Villafane, J. H., Capra, F.,

Guccione, A. A., & PIlastrini, P. (2013). Effect of therapeutic exercise on pain and disability in the management of chronic nonspecific neck pain: systematic review and meta-analysis of randomized trials. *Physical Therapy, 93*(8), 1026-36.

[23] Busch, A. J., Barber, K. A. R., Overend, T. J., Peloso, P. M. J., & Schachter, C. L. (2007). Exercise for treating fibromyalgia syndrome. Cochrane Database of Systematic Reviews. (4), Art. No.: CD003786.-See more at: http://summaries.cochrane.org/CD003786/MUSKEL_exercise-for-fibromyalgia#sthash.bwIlSsp2.dpuf

[24] Goodman, A. (2014). Aerobic Exercise "most effective weapon" for fibromyalgia. http://www.medscape.com/viewarticle/827054.

[25] Kennedy, N. (2006). Exercise therapy for patients with rheumatoid arthritis: safety of intensive programmes and effects upon bone mineral density and disease activity: a literature review. *Physical Therapy Reviews, 11*, 263-268.

[26] Uthman, O., van der Windt, D., Jordan, J., Dziedzic, K., Healey, E., Peat, G., & Foster, N. (2013). Exercise for lower limb osteoarthritis: systematic review incorporating trial sequential analysis and network meta-analysis. *British Medical Journal*, 347, f5555.

[27] *Tufts University Health & Nutrition Newsletter*. August 2003 Supplement.

[28] White, D. K., Tudor-Locke, C., Ahnag, Y., Fielding, R., LaValley, M., Felson DT . . . Neogi, T. (2014). Daily walking and the risk of incident functional limitation in knee osteoarthritis: an observational study. *Arthritis Care Research, 66*(9), 1328-36.

[29] Shnayderman, I. & Katz-Leurer, M. (2013). An aerobic walking programme versus muscle strengthening programme for chronic low-back pain: a randomized controlled trial. *Clinical Rehabilitation*, (3), 207-14.

[30] De Vierville, J. (1997). A history of aquatic rehabilitation. In: *Comprehensive Aquatic Rehabilitation, First Edition*, Becker B. E., C. A. (ed). Newton, MA: Butterworth-Heineman.

[31] De Vierville, J. (2004). Aquatic rehabilitation: a historical perspective, In: *Comprehensive Aquatic Rehabilitation*, 2nd edition. Cole, A. J., B.B. (ed.). Philadelphia, PA: Betterworth Heineman, 1-18.

[32] Kinnaird, D. W. & Becker, B. (2008). *Contemporary Aquatic Therapy and Pain Management in Integrative Pain Management*. Audette, J. & Bailey A. (eds.). Humana Press, 285-306.

[33] Franklin D. Roosevelt Presidential Library and Museum. Roosevelt Facts and Figures. http://www.fdrlibrary.marist.edu/facts/.

[34] Altan, L., Bingol, U., Aykac, M., Loc, Z., & Yurtkuran, M. (2004). Investigation of the effects of pool-based exercise on fibromyalgia syndrome. *Rheumatology International, 24*(5), 272-77.

[35] Ariyoshi, M, Sonoda, K., Nagata, K., Mashima, T., Zenmyo, M., Paku, C. . . . Mutoh Y. (1999). Efficacy of aquatic exercises for patients with low-back pain. *The Karume Medical Journal, 46*(2), 91-96.

[36] LeFort, S. M. & Hannah, T. E. (1994). Return to work following an aquafitness and muscle strengthening program for the low back injured. *Archives of Physical Medicine and Rehabilitation, 75*(11), 1247-1255.

[37] Fishman, L. & Satonstall, E. (2008). *Yoga in Pain Management in Integrative Pain Management*, Audette, J. & Bailey, A. (eds.) Humana Press, 259-260.

[38] Mamtani. R. & Frishman, W. (2008). *Ayurveda and Yoga in Complementary and Alternative Medicine in Pain Management*, Weintraub, M., Mamtani, R., & Micozzi, M. (eds.) Springer Publishing Company, 259.

[39] Fishman. (2008). *Yoga in Pain Management*, 62.

[40] Posadzki, P., Emst, E., Tery, R., & Lee, M. S. (2011). Is yoga effective for pain? A systematic review of randomized clinical trials. *Complementary Therapies in Medicine, 19*(5), 281-7.

[41] Williams, K. A., Petronis, J., Smith, D., Goodrich, D., Wu, J., Ravi, N., Doyle, E. J., Jr., Gregory Juckett, R., Minoz Kolar, M., Gross, R., & Steinberg, L. (2005). Effect of Iyengar yoga therapy for chronic low-back pain. *Pain, 115*(1-2), 107-117.

[42] Monro, R., Bhardwaj, A. K., Gupta, R. K., Telles, S., Allen, B., & Little, P. (2014). Disc extrusions and bulges in nonspecific low-back pain and sciatica: Exploratory randomised controlled trial comparing yoga therapy and normal medical treatment. *Journal of Back and Musculoskeletal Rehabilitation*, 2014 September 29 (Epub ahead of print) http://www.ncbi.nlm.nih.gov/pubmed/25271201

[43] Mamtani & Fisherman. (2008). *Ayurveda and Yoga*, 279.

[44] Mamatani & Fisherman. (2008). *Ayurveda and Yoga.* 263-4.

Chp. 10: Homeopathy (pp. 171–179)

[1] Chickcramane, P.S., Suresh, A. K., Bellare, J. R., & Kane, S. G. (2010). Extreme homeopathic dilutions retain starting materials: A nanopathic perspective. *Homeopathy.* 99(4), 231-42.

[2] Robins, Natalie. (2005). *Copeland's Cure: Homeopathy and the War Between Conventional and Alternative Medicine,* New York. Alfred A. Knopf, 6.

[3] Robins. (2005). *Copeland's Cure,* 7.

[4] Robins. (2005). *Copeland's Cure,* 7.

[5] Robins. (2005). *Copeland's Cure,* 18.

[6] Zell, J., Connert, W. D., Mau, J., & Feurstake, G. (1989). Treatment of Acute Sprains of the Ankle: A Controlled Double-Blind Trial to Test the Effectiveness of a Homeopathic Ointment. *Biological Therapy, VII*(1), 1-6.

[7] Schneider, C. (2011). Traumeel–an emerging option to nonsteroidal anti-inflammatory drugs in the management of acute musculoskeletal injuries. *International Journal of General Medicine, 4,* 225-34.

[8] http://en.wikipedia.org/wiki/Regulation_and_prevalence_of_homeopathy#United_States accessed on 11/2/14.

[9] Hershoff, A. (1996). *Homeopathy for Musculoskeletal Healing.* North Atlantic Books.

[10] Henderson M., (2007, May 23). Hard-up NHS trusts cut back on unproven homeopathy treatment. *The Times.*

[11] The end of homeopathy. (2005). *The Lancet,* 366(9487), 690.

[12] Shang, A. et al. (2005). Are the clinical effects of homoeopathy placebo effects? Comparative study of placebo-controlled trials of homoeopathy and allopathy, *The Lancet, 366*(9487), 690.

[13] Shang, A. et al. (2005). Are the clinical effects of homoeopathy placebo effects?

[14] Letter written by Prof. Michael Baum et al., May 19, 2006.

[15] Royals favoured hospital at risk as homeopathy backlash gathers pace. (2007, April 8). *The Observer.*

[16] Royals favoured hospital at risk as homeopathy backlash gathers pace.

(2007).

[17] Homeopathy: Tinctures or a trick of the mind, (2010, February 26).*The Independent.*

[18] Homeopathy: Tinctures or a trick of the mind, (2010, February 26).*The Independent.*

[19] Gibson, R. G., Gibson, S. L. M., MacNeill, A. D., & Buchanan, W. W. (1980). Homeopathic therapy in rheumatoid arthritis evaluation by double-blind clinical therapeutic trial. *British Journal of Clinical Pharmacology, 9*, 453-459

[20] Brigo, B. (1987). Le traitement homeopathique de la migraine: une otude de 60 cas, controlee en double aveugle. *Journal of Liga Medicorum Homoeopathica Internationalis*, 18-25 reprinted in English in *The Berlin Journal on Research in Homeopathy* March 1991, 1(2), 98-106.

[21] Shealy, C. N., Thomlinson, P. R., Cox, R. H., & Bormeyer, V. (1998). Osteoarthritis Pain: A Comparison of Homoeopathy and Acetaminophen. *American Journal of Pain Management, 8*, 89-91.

[22] Bell, I. R., Lewis, II D. A., Brooks, A. J., Schwartz, G. E., Lewis, S. E., Walsh, B. T., Baldwin, & C. M. (2004). Improved clinical status in fibromyalgia patients treated with individualized homeopathic remedies versus placebo. *Rheumatology Advance Access.* http://rheumatology.oupjournals.org/cgi/reprint/keh111 accessed on 11/1/14.

[23] Beer, A. M., Fey, S., Zimmer, M., Teske, W., Schremmer, D., & Wiebelitz, K. R. (2012). Effectiveness ad safety of a homeopathic drug combination in the treatment of chronic low-back pain. A double-blind, randomrized, placebo-controlled clinical trial. *MMW Fortschritte der Medizin, 154* Suppl 2:48-57.

[24] Boehm, K., Raak, C., Cramer, H., Lauche, R., & Ostermann, T. (2014). Homeopathy in the treatment of fibromyalgia—a comprehensive literature-review and meta-analysis. *Complementary Therapies in Medicine, 22*, 731-742.

Chp. 11: Acupuncture (pp. 181–186)

[1] Wang, D. & Audette, J. (2008). Acupuncture in Pain Management in *Contemporary Pain Medicine: Integrative Pain Medicine: The Science and Practice of Complementary and Alternative Medicine in Pain Management*, Audette JF and Bailey A, eds. Totowa, NJ:

Humana Press, 379.

[2] Wang & Audette. (2008). *Acupuncture in Pain Management*, 380-83.

[3] Wang & Audette. (2008). *Acupuncture in Pain Management*, 383.

[4] Reston, J. (1971). Now, about my operation in Peking. *The New York Times*.

[5] Wikipedia, Miriam Lee. http://en.wikipedia.org/wiki/Miriam_Lee and History, California Acupuncture Board. http://www.acupuncture.ca.gov/about_us/history.shtml on 3/21/15.

[6] National Certification Commission for Acupuncture and Oriental Medicine State Licensing Requirements List. http://mx.nccaom.org/StateLicensing.aspx on 3/21/15.

[7] Barnes, P. M., Bloom, B., & Nahin, R. L. (2008). Complementary and Alternative medicine use among adults and children: United States, 2007. *Natl Health Stat Report*. (12):1-23.

[8] Sherman, K. J., Cherkin, D. C., Eisenberg, D. M, Erro, J., Hrbek, A., & Deyo, R, A. (2005). The practice of acupuncture: who are the providers and what do they do? *Annals of Family Medicine*, *3*(2), 151-158.

[9] Sherman et al. (2005). The practice of acupuncture.

[10] Sherman et al. (2005). The practice of acupuncture.

[11] Cherkin, D. C., Deyo, R. A., Sherman, K. J., et al. Characteristics of licensed acupuncturists, chiropractors, massage therapists, and naturopathic physicians. *J Am Board Fam Pract,15* 378-390

[12] Sherman et al. (2005). The practice of acupuncture.

[13] Wang & Audette. (2008). Acupuncture in Pain Management, 385-388

[14] Wang & Audette. (2008). Acupuncture in Pain Management, 389-391.

[15] Wang & Audette. (2008). Acupuncture in Pain Management, 396

[16] Hopton, A. & MacPherson, H. (2010). Acupuncture for chronic pain: Is acupuncture more than an effective placebo? A systematic review of pooled data from meta-analyses. *Pain Practice, 10*(2), 94-102.

[17] Vickers, A., Cronin, A., Maschino, A., Lewith, G., MacPherson, H., Victor, N., Foster, N., Sherman, K., Witt, C., & Linde, K. (2012). Acupuncture for chronic pain: individual patient data meta-analysis. *Archives of Internal Medicine, 172*(9), 1444-1453.

[18] Haake, M., Muller, H., Schade-Brittinger, C., Basler, H., Schafer H, Maier C, Endres H, Trampisch H, Molsberger A. (2007). German acupuncture trials (GERAC) for chronic low-back pain. *Archives of Internal Medicine, 167*(17), 1892-1898.

[19] Deare, JC,, Zheng, Z, Xue, CCL, Liu, JP, Shang, J, Scott, SW, & Littlejohn, G. (2013). Acupuncture for fibromyalgia. *Cochrane Review.*
http://www.cochrane.org//CD007070/MUSKEL_acupuncture-for-fibromyalgia on 3/15/15.

[20] World Health Organization. (2002). Acupuncture review and analysis of reports on controlled clinical trials, 5.

[21] Personal interview.

Chp. 12: Energy Healing (pp. 187–193)

[1] Leskowitz E. (2008). Therapeutic touch. In *Complementary and Integrative Medicine in Pain Management*, Wintraub M, Mamtani R and Micozzi M, Editors. Springer Publishing Company, 163-174.

[2] http://en.wikipedia.org/wiki/Therapeutic_touch accessed on 4/5/15.

[3] Jhaveri A, Walsh SJ, Wang Y, McCarthy M, Gronowisz G. (2008). Therapeutic touch affects DNA synthesis and mineralization of human osteoblasts in culture. *Journal of Orthopedic Research.*(11), 1541-6.

[4] Personal interview

[5] Emily's Little Experiment, (1998, April 13). *TIME.*

[6] A Closer Look at Therapeutic Touch, Rosa, Linda, Rosa, Emily et. al, (1998). *Journal of the American Medical Association, 279*(13).

[7] Kolata, G. (1998, April 3). A child's paper poses a medical challenge. *New York Times.*

[8] Cox, T. (2003). A nurse-statistician reanalyzes data from the Rosa therapeutic touch study. *Alternative Therapies, 9*(1), 58-64.

[9] http://en.wikipedia.org/wiki/Stephen_Barrett

[10] Cox. (2003). A nurse statistician reanalyzes . . .

[11] Winstead-Fry, P & Kijek J. (1999). An integrative review and meta-analysis of therapeutic touch research. *Alternative Therapies in Health and Medicine,* (6):58-67.

[12] So, PS, Jiang, Y, Qin, Y. (2008). Touch therapies for pain relief in adults. *Cochrane Database of Systemic Reviews*, 8;(4).

[13] Hammerschlag, R., Marx, B., & Aickin, M. Nontouch Biofield. (2014) Therapy: A Systematic Review of Human Randomized Controlled Trials Reporting Use of Only Nonphysical Contact Treatment. *The Journal of Alternative and Complementary Medicine, 20*(12), 881-892,

[14] Ananth, S. (2006). "Health Forum 2005 Complementary and Alternative Medicine Survey of Hospitals." News release, American Hospital Association.

Chp. 13: Marijuana (pp. 195–207)

[1] Snyder, S. H. (1970, December 13). What we have forgotten about pot. *New York Times Magazine*.

[2] Sloman, L. (1979). *The History of Marijuana in America: Reefer Madness*, 26.

[3] Nicoll, R. & Alger B. (2004, December). The brain's own marijuana. *Scientific American*, 70.

[4] Nicoll & Alger. (2004). The brain's own marijuana.

[5] *The La Guardia Committee Report: The Marihuana Problem in the City of New York*. (1994). Mayor's Committee on Marihuana, by the New York Academy of Medicine, City of New York. http://www.druglibrary.org/schaffer/library/studies/lag/lagmenu.ht m on April 25 2015.

[6] Bonnie, R., Whitebread II. (1974). *The Marijuana Conviction: A History of Marihuana Prohibition in the United States*, 117.

[7] Grinspoon, L. (1994). *Marijuana Reconsidered*, 2nd ed, Harvard University Press, 14.

[8] Storrs, C. (2009, November 17). The AMA eases its stance on marijuana. *Scientific American*.

[9] Harris, G. (2006, April 21). FDA dismisses medical benefit from marijuana. *New York Times*, A1.

[10] Harris. (2006). FDA dismisses medical benefit from marijuana.

[11] Harris. (2006). FDA dismisses medical benefit from marijuana.

[12] Stern, R. & DiFonzo, J. H. (2009). The End of the Red Queen's Race: Medical Marijuana in the New Century. *Quinnipiac Law Review*,

27, 707.

[13] The Institute of Medicine. (1999). *Marijuana and Medicine: Assessing the Science Base.*

[14] WebMD. Marinol. Side effects. http://www.webmd.com/drugs/drug-9308-marinol+Oral.aspx?drugid=9308&drugname=Marinol+Oral&page number=6 accessed on May 3, 2015.

[15] Issa, M. A., Narang, S., Jamison, R. N., et al. (2014). The subjective psychoactive effects of oral dronabinol studied in a randomized controlled crossover clinical trial for pain. *Clinical Journal of Pain, 30,* 472-478

[16] ProCon.org. 10 pharmaceutical drugs based on cannabis.http://medicalmarijuana.procon.org/view.resource.php?re sourceID=000883 on 4/25/15.

[17] ProCon.org. 10 pharmaceutical drugs based on cannabis.

[18] Mehmedic, Z., Chandra, S., Slade, D., et al. (2010). Potency trends of 9-THC and other cannabinoids in confiscated cannabis preparations from 1993 to 2008. *Journal of Forensic Science, 55,* 1209-1217.

[19] Nicoll & Alger. (2004). The brain's own marijuana

[20] Mackie, K. (2006). Cannabinoid receptors as therapeutic targets. *Annual Review of Pharmacology and Toxicology, 46,* 101-22.

[21] Mackie. (2006). Cannabinoid receptors as therapeutic targets.

[22] Nicole & Alger. (2004). The brain's own marijuana.71-72.

[23] Pertwee, R. G. (2006). The pharmacology of cannabinoid receptors and their ligans: an overview. *International Journal of Obesity, 30*(S14).

[24] Nicoll & Alger. (2004). The brain's own marijuana, 74-75.

[25] Grinspoon. (1994). *Marijuana Reconsidered,* 153.

[26] Grinspoon, L. (2006, May 5). Puffing is the best medicine. *LA Times,* B13.

[27] Grinspoon. (2006). Puffing is the best medicine.

[28] Lynch, M. & Campbell, F. (2011). Cannabinoids for treatment of chronic non-cancer pain; a systematic review of randomized trials. *British Journal of Clinical Pharmacology, 72*(5), 735-44.

[29] Boychuk, D., Goddard, G., Mauro, G., & Orellan, M. (2015). The Effectiveness of Cannabinoids in the management of chronic nonmalignant neuropathic pain: a systematic review. *Journal of Oral & Facial Pain and Headache, 29*(1), 7-14.

[30] Webb, C. W. & Webb, S. M. (2014). Therapeutic benefits of cannabis: a patient survey. *Hawai'i Journal of Medicine and Public Health, 73*(4), 109-11.

[31] Burgdorf, J. R., Kilmer, B., & Pacula, R. L. (2011). Heterogeneity in the composition of marijuana seized in California. *Drug and Alcohol Dependence,* 117:59-61

[32] Niesink, R. J. & van Laar, M. W. (2013) Does cannabidiol protect against adverse psychological effects of THC? *Frontiers in Psychiatry, 4,* 130.

[33] Schatman, M. E. (2015). Medical marijuana: The state of the science. Medscape. http://www.medscape.com/viewarticle/839155 on May 3.

[34] Schatman. (2015). Medical marijuana.

[35] Malik, A. & D'Souza, D. C. (2006).Gone to pot: the association between cannabis and psychosis. *Psychiatric Times,* 23, 28.

[36] Editorial. Dangerous habits. Lancet, 1 http://www.ncbi.nlm.nih.gov/pmc/articles/PMC1853086/998, 352:1565.

[37] Editorial. Dangerous habits. *Lancet,* 1.

[38] Earleywine, M. & Barnwell, S.M. (2007). Decreased respiratory symptoms in cannabis users who vaporize. *Harm Reduction Journal,* 4:11. http://www.ncbi.nlm.nih.gov/pmc/articles/PMC1853086/ on 5/24/15.

[39] Kaufman, M. (2006, May 26). Study finds no cancer-marijuana connection. *Washington Post,* A3.

[40] Munson, A. E. et al.(1975). Anticancer activity of cannabinoids. *Journal of the National Cancer Institute,* 55, 597.

[41] Munson. (1975). Anticancer activity of cannabinoids.

[42] US Department of Health and Human Services, Public Health Servics, National Institutes of Health. (1995). NTF Technical Report on the Toxicology and Carcinogenesis Studies of 1-Trans-Delta9-

Tetrahydrocannabinol in F344/N Rats and B6C3F1 Mice (Gavage Studies). Washington, D.C., 1994:7.

[43] "Marijuana's Active Ingredient Shown to Inhibit Primary Marker of Alzheimer's Disease." (2006, August 9). The Scripps Research Institute. Press release.

[44] Werner C. (2011). *Marijuana, Gateway to Health: How Cannabis Protects US from Cancer and Alzheimer's Disease.* San Francisco: Dachstar Press.

[45] Wener. (2011). *Marijuana, Gateway to Health.*

[46] Hall, W. & Solowij, N. (1998). Adverse effects of cannabis. *Lancet,* 353, 1611.

[47] Cichewicz, D. L., Martin, Z. L., Smith, F.L., & Welch, S.P. (1999). Enhancement of mu opioid antinociception by oral delta9-tetrahydrocannabinol: Dose-response analysis and receptor identification. *Journal of Pharmacology and Experimental Therapeutics, 289*(2), 859–67.

[48] Cichewicz, D. L. & Welch, S. P. (2003). Modulation of oral morphine antinociceptive tolerance and naloxone-precipitated withdrawal signs by oral delta9-tetrahydrocannabinol. *The Journal of Pharmacology and Experimental Therapeutics,* 305, 812-817.

[49] Reiman, A. (2009). Cannabis as a substitute for alcohol and other drugs. *Harm Reduction Journal, 6*(35). http://www.harmreductionjournal.com/content/6/1/35 on 5/26/15.

[50] Bachhuber, M. A, Saloner, B., Cunningham, C. O, & Barry, C. L. (2014). Medical cannabis laws and opioid analgesic overdose mortality in the United States, 1999-2010. *JAMA Internal Medicine, 144*(10), 1668-73.

[51] ProCon.org. 23 legal medical marijuana states and DC. Updated November 30, 2014. http://medicalmarijuana.procon.org/view.resource.php?resourceID=000881.

[52] Controlled Substances Act, 21 U.S.C. Sections 801-971 (2000).

[53] 21 U.S.C. Section 812(b)(1) (2000).

[54] Stern & DiFonzo, 711.

[55] Stern & DiFonzo, 719.

[56] Gonzales v. Raich, 545 US 1 (2005).

[57] Stern & DeFonzo, 719.

[58] Stern & DeFonzo, 721.

[59] Santa Cruz, 279 F. Supp. 2d.

[60] Buchana, W. (2008, February 7). Pot dispensaries shut in response to federal threat. *San Francisco Chronicle*, B1.

[61] Stern & DiFonzo, 673-765.

[62] Frellick, M. (2014, December 22). Feds can no longer raid state medical marijuana dispensaries. Medscape. http://www.medscape.com/viewarticle/837011 on April 26, 2015.

[63] Elders, J. (2008, March 28) Former Surgeon General: Mainstream medicine has endorsed medical marijuana. Alternet. http://www.alternet.org/story/80582/former_surgeon_general%3A _mainstream_medicine_has_endorsed_medical_marijuana on April 26, 2015.

[64] Procon.org. Votes and polls. http://medicalmarijuana.procon.org/view.additional-resource.php?resourceID=000151 on April 26, 2015

[65] Procon.org. Votes and polls. http://medicalmarijuana.procon.org/view.additional-resource.php?resourceID=000151 on April 26, 2015

[66] Healy, J. (2015, June 15). Workers can be fired for marijuana use, Colorado court rules. *New York Times*.

[67] Dietrich, A. & McDaniel, W. F. (2004). Endocannabinoids and exercise. *British Journal of Sports Medicine*, 38:536-541.

Chp. 14: Low Level Laser Therapy (pp. 209–216)

[1] Huang, Y. Y., Chen, A. C., Carroll, J. D., & Hamblin, M. R. (2009). Biphasic dose response in low level light therapy. *Dose Response,* 7(4):358-83.

[2] Huang et al. (2009). Biphasic dose response.

[3] Merrick, R. V., Kahn, F., & Saraga, F. (2013) Treatment of postherpetic neuralgia with low level laser therapy. *Practical Pain Management*. http://www.practicalpainmanagement.com/treatments/complement ary/lasers/treatment-postherpetic-neuralgia-low-level-laser-therapy

on 8/15/15.

[4] http://www.thorlaser.com/downloads/brochures/THOR-Brochure-web.pdf accessed on 8/15/15.

[5] Aimbire, F., Albertini, R., Pacheco, M. T., Castro-Faria-Neto, H. C., Leonardo, P. S., Iversen, V, Lopes-Martins, R. A., & Bjordal, J, M. (2006) Low-level laser therapy induces dose-dependent reduction of TNFalpha levels in acute inflammation. *Photomedicine and Laser Surgery, 24*, 33-7.

[6] Goncalves, W. L., Souza, F. M., Conti, C. L., Cirqueira, J. P., Rocha, W. A, Pires, J. G., Barros, L. A., & Moyses MR. (2007). Influence of He-Ne laser therapy on the dynamics of wound healing in mice treated with anti-inflammatory drugs. *Brazilian Journal of Medical and Biological Research*, 40:877-84.

[7] Chow, R. T., Johnson, M. I., Lopes-Martins, R. A., & Bjordal, J. M. (2009). Efficacy of low-level laser therapy in the management of neck pain: a systematic review and meta-analysis of randomised placebo or active-treatment controlled trials. *Lancet, 374*(9705), 1897-908.

[8] Fulop, A. M., Dhimmer, S., Deluca, J. R., Johanson, D. D., Lenz, R. V., Patel, K. B., et al. (2010). A meta-analysis of the efficacy of laser phototherapy on pain relief. *Clinical Journal of Pain, 26*, 729–736.

[9] Haslerud, S., Magnussen, L., Joensen, J., Alvaro, R., Lopes-Martins, B., & Bjordai, J. M. (2015). The efficacy of low-level laser therapy for shoulder tendinopathy: A systematic review and meta-analysis of randomized controlled trials. *Physiotherapy Research International, 20*(2), 108-25.

[10] Law, D., MDonough, S., Bleakley, C., Baxter, G. D., & Tuity, S. (2015). Laser acupuncture for treating musculoskeletal pain: a systematic review with meta-analysis. *Journal of Acupuncture Meridian Studies, 8(*1), 2-16.

[11] Chen, J., Huang, Z., Ge, M., & Gao, M. (2015). Efficacy of low-level laser therapy in the treatment of TMDs: a meta-analysis of 14 randomised controlled trials. *Journal of Oral Rehabiitation, 42*(4):291-9.

[12] Ip D, Fu NY. (2015). Can intractable discogenic back pain be managed by low-level laser therapy without recourse to operative intervention? *Journal of Pain Research, 8*, 253-6.

[13] Harkess, L. B., DeLelis, S., Carnegie, D. H., & Burke, J. (2006). Improved foot sensitivity and pain reduction in patients with peripheral neuropathy after treatment with monochromatic infrared photo energy--MIRE. *Journal of Diabetes Complications, 20*(2), 81-7.

[14] Powell, M. W., Carnegie, D. H. & Burke, T. J. (2006). Reversal of diabetic peripheral neuropathy with phototherapy (MIRE) decreases falls and the fear of falling and improves activities of daily living in seniors. *Age and Ageing.* (1), 11-6

[15] Containdications for use of therapeutic laser. (2010). *Practical Pain Management.*
http://www.practicalpainmanagement.com/treatments/complement ary/lasers/contraindications-use-therapeutic-laser on 8/15/15.

[16] Personal interview.

[17] http://www.fda.gov/Radiation-mittingProducts/ResourcesforYouRadiationEmittingProducts/ucm 252761.htm#5 accessed on 8/15/15.

[18] http://www.udel.edu/PT/PT%20Clinical%20Services/journalclub/caserou nds/11-12/September/MedicalCoverageAntiLaser.pdf accessed on 8/15/15.

[19] http://www.aetna.com/cpb/medical/data/300_399/0363.html accessed on 8/15/15

[20] https://www.bcbsms.com/index.php?q=provider-medical-policy-search.html&action=viewPolicy&path=%2Fpolicy%2Femed%2FL ow+Level+Laser+Therapy+as+a+Treatment+of+Carpal+Tunnel+S yndrome.html accessed on 8/15/15.

[21] https://www.cms.gov/medicare-coverage-database/details/nca-decision-memo.aspx?NCAId=176&ver=24&NcaName=Infrared+Therapy+ Devices&SearchType=Advanced&CoverageSelection=Both&NCS election=NCA%7CCAL%7CNCD%7CMEDCAC%7CTA%7CM CD&ArticleType=Ed%7CKey%7CSAD%7CFAQ&PolicyType=F inal&s=5%7C6%7C66%7C67%7C9%7C38%7C63%7C41%7C64 %7C65%7C44&KeyWord=low+level+laser+therapy&KeyWordL ookUp=Doc&KeyWordSearchType=Exact&kq=true&bc=IAAAA CAAEAAA& accessed on 8/15/15.

Chp. 15: Multidisciplinary Programs (pp. 217–219)

[1] International Association for the Study of Pain. (2012*). Pain Clinical*

Updates, 20(7), 1.

[2] Flor, H., Fydrich, T. & Turk, D. C. (1992). Efficacy of multidisciplinary pain treatment centers: a meta-analytic review. *Pain, 49*(2), 221-30.

[3] Guzman, J., Esmail, R., Karjalainen, K., Malmivaara, A., Irvin, E., & Bombardiar, C. (2001). Mutidisciplinary rehabilitation for chronic low-back pain: systematic review. *BMJ, 322,* 1515.

[4] Patrick, L. E., Altmaier, E. M., & Found, E, M. (2004). Long-term outcomes in multidisciplinary treatment of chronic low-back pain: results of a 13-year follow-up. *Spine,* 29(8), 850-5.

[5] Meir, B. (2013). *A World of Hurt: Fixing Pain Medicine's Biggest Mistake,* Kindle Single.

[6] Anooshian, J., Streltzer, J. & Goebert, D. (1999). Effectiveness of a psychiatric pain clinic. *Psychosomatics,* 40, 226–32.

[7] Jeffery, M. M., Butler M, Stark A, Kane RL. *Multidisciplinary pain programs for chronic noncancer pain.* Rockville, MD: Agency for Healthcare Research and Quality; 2011

[8] Schatman M, (2012). Interdisciplinary Chronic Pain Management: International Perspectives. *Pain Clinic Updates,* International Association for the Study of Pain, XX(7), 1-5.

[9] Marketdata Enterprises. (1995). *Chronic Pain Management Programs: A Market Analysis.* New York: Valley Stream.

[10] National Center for Health Statistics. (1997). National Hospital Discharge Survey Series 13(144), Washington, DC, US Department of Health and Human Services, Center for Disease Control.

[11] Bell, G., Kidd, D., & North, R. (1997). Cost-effectiveness analysis of spinal cord stimulation in treatment of failed back surgery syndrome. *Journal of Pain Symptom Management,* 13, 286-295.

[12] Committee on Advancing Pain Research, Care and Education; Institute of Medicine. (2011). *Relieving Pain in America: A Blueprint for Transforming Prevention, Care, Education, and Research.* The National Academies Press, 4.

Chp. 16: The Pain Treatment Parity Act (pp. 221–225)

[1] Based on the Consumer Price Index Inflation Calculator 1980-2015. http://data.bls.gov/cgi-bin/cpicalc.pl.

ACKNOWLEDGEMENTS

I am extremely grateful to all the medical pioneers who defied conventional thinking and explored safer and more effective therapies. They taught me to look at healing in a different way, helped me to heal myself, and ultimately led me to write this book. Norman Cousins, Dr. Bernie Siegel, Louise Hay, Dr. Deepak Chopra, Dr. Andrew Weil, Dr. Joseph Mercola, Andrew Saul, PhD, Belleruth Naperstek, Jon Kabat Zinn, Dr. Howard Schubiner, Roger Callahan, PhD, Stu Donaldson, PhD, and many others influenced me tremendously.

I also want to thank the many medical providers who contributed to my own healing, especially psychologist Marty Leyden, who introduced me to biofeedback; Rolfers David Delaney and Allan Davidson; Mary Sise, LCSW, who introduced me to Thought Field Therapy; and Dr. Ann Tobin, a holistic physician who has provided me with general medical guidance for many years.

This book would not have been possible without the many patients, medical providers, and other experts who shared their experiences and wisdom with me, including Dr. Norman Marcus, Dr. Robert Verkerk, Dr. Philomena Kong, Sheryl Drake, DC, Lee Masterson, DC, Michelle Kelleher, PT, John Grazione, PT, Dick Marrone, PT, Susan Antelis, LMHC and many others. Beth Eisman and Chris Graf provided research support and Dionne Leigh and Amy Buchanan provided secretarial support. Violeta Damjanovic designed the book cover. Photographer Oscar Aguirre took my picture for the back cover. Thanks also to my editor Hannah Eason.

I also greatly appreciate the many friends, colleagues and clients who encouraged me and cheered me on along the way.

INDEX

A

abdominal muscles 163
abdominal pain 36, 66–8, 245
abdominal surgery 214
abnormalities 23, 52, 55, 72–3, 120, 162–63
abuse 18, 20, 22, 30, 53, 63, 76, 129, 203, 221, 230, 231–32, 234, 243, 249
  abuse-deterrent 20, 26
  abuse-prevention 24
  abuse-resistant 25, 234
acetaminophen 24, 31, 33, 37–8, 153, 179, 236, 268
acupoints 181
acupressure 104, 248
acupuncture 2, 8, 11, 49, 80–1, 104, 181–87, 211, 223, 252, 258, 268, 269, 276
  acupuncture points 81, 181, 183, 211
  acupuncturists 48, 144, 183, 224, 269
addiction 6, 18–20, 22, 23–6, 29–31, 33, 64, 146, 195, 221–22, 232–33
Agency for Health Care Policy and Research 88, 228, 249–51
alcohol 22, 37, 48, 53, 202, 236, 272, 274
  alcohol dependence 272
  alcohol exposure 37
  alcohol problems 48
Alexander, Caleb 20
Alliance for Natural Health 124, 127, 130–31, 257
American Medical Association 88–9, 90, 173, 192, 195–96, 229, 270–71
American Physical Therapy Association 99, 100, 251
anterior cingulate cortex (ACC) 62

anti-inflammatory 17, 33, 36, 88, 113, 119, 150, 155, 158, 178, 209, 235, 253–54, 276
  anti-inflammatory drugs 17, 33, 36, 88, 119, 178, 235, 253, 276
  anti-inflammatory effects 150, 155
antidepressants 9, 17–18, 21, 47, 73, 116, 154, 228–29
antioxidants 111–12, 123
anxiety 10, 21-2, 24, 41, 52, 61, 65, 68, 80-2, 104-6, 154, 198, 200, 245, 248
aquafitness 265
arthritis 1, 35, 40, 67, 113, 145, 151–57, 163, 165, 171, 178, 199, 237, 255, 260–62, 264–65, 267
aspartame 142, 145–46, 258–59
aspirin 17, 24, 33–4, 36–8, 235
AstraZeneca 10
autism 37, 38, 236
  autism epidemic 236
  autistic 236
Ayurvedic 187

B

Barber, Joseph 82, 249
barbiturates 114
Barrett, Stephen 192, 270
beta-carotene 134
Bextra 39
biofeedback 10, 14, 61, 67–74, 84, 183, 187, 217, 223, 229, 244–46, 279
  biofeedback practitioner 70, 73
blood flow 61–7, 245
blood pressure 10, 61, 83
blood sugar 146
blood supply 108, 147
bloodletting 172
bloodstream 118

body-based practices 87–9, 91, 93, 95, 97, 99, 101, 103, 105, 107, 109, 249

bodywork 2, 101–03, 105, 252, 254

boswellia 151, 152, 259, 260

brain 13–15, 23–4, 30, 61–3, 67, 72–3, 75, 81, 172, 183, 198, 200, 210, 234, 242–45

  brain abnormalities 23

  brain activity 15, 183

  brain damage 172

  brain mapping 73

  brain regions 61, 73

  brain wave 14, 67, 72

butterbur 152–53, 260

C

California 24, 25, 91, 182, 200, 201, 203–04, 250, 268, 272

cancer 1, 13, 28, 30, 54, 116, 123, 142, 145, 151, 171, 189, 196–97, 201, 202, 204, 228, 240, 273

  cancer institute 201, 273

  cancer pain 197, 228, 231, 238, 272

  cancer-marijuana 273

  cancerous 213

  carcinogenesis 273

cardiovascular 36, 115–16, 158, 200, 236

Carragee, Eugene 55, 239

Carroll, James 213

cat's claw 153, 261

celiac 142, 143, 144, 258

Celebrex 11, 17, 36–9, 157, 236, 262

Centers for Disease Control (CDC) 31, 227, 231, 234–35

chemotherapy 196–97

chiropractic 12, 36, 69, 87–9, 90–4, 96, 106, 186, 216, 223, 249–51

  chiropractic manipulation 106, 249

chiropractic profession 87, 88, 90, 250
chiropractic treatment 69, 87–8, 91–2, 96
chiropractic visits 92–3
chiropractors 5, 48, 81, 87–94, 101, 222, 224, 250, 269
clinical conditions 183, 205
clinical effects 175, 267
clinical evidence 7
clinical interventions 262
clinical journal 211, 237, 256, 271, 276
clinical outcomes 241, 252
clinical pharmacology 260, 272
clinical psychology 3, 247
clinical trials 7, 39, 52, 125, 168, 178, 192, 211, 266, 269
Cochrane Database 18, 41, 66, 104, 164, 184, 192, 231, 237, 253, 264
Codex 140–41
co-pay 92, 96, 99–100
Corral, Valery 204
cortisol 183, 243, 248
curcumin 155, 156, 261, 262

D

Davidson, Allan 106, 253, 279
death 2, 20, 21, 22, 24–5, 36–7, 39–40, 44, 202, 204, 232
death worldwide from cannabis 202
death, Heath Ledger 22
death, Michael Jackson 21
death, Philip Seymour Hoffman 22
deaths 19, 24, 29, 35, 37, 38, 173, 202, 214
   deaths associated with opioids 30
   deaths attributed to Vioxx 38
   deaths from liver failure 37
   deaths from opioid overdose 19

Delaney, David 107, 279

depression 9, 32, 52, 65, 80, 81, 82, 104–06, 115, 117, 142, 158, 165, 179, 200, 229, 248

desensitization 77–79, 246–48
  desensitization and reprocessing 77, 247
  desensitization in fibromyalgia 247
  desensitization in psychotherapy 248

diabetes 1, 40–1 116–17, 156, 212, 214–15, 256, 262, 276.

diet 47, 111–12, 120–21, 130, 132, 134, 137, 139, 141, 142, 144, 145–46, 255, 259

dietary supplements 127, 141, 195, 258

disorders 14, 32, 62, 66, 87, 115–16, 143, 153–55, 211–12, 214, 240, 248

Domenici, Pete 222

dopamine 24, 183

dorsolateral prefrontal cortex (DLPFC) 62

Drake, Sheryl 93–4, 279

drugs 6, 9, 12, 16–23, 27–33, 36–7, 40–1, 44, 88–9, 114, 119, 124, 127, 129, 131–32, 143, 149–50, 154, 177–78, 184, 196, 202, 206, 217, 229, 232, 235–36, 238, 253–54, 258, 267, 271–72, 274, 276
  drugmakers 19, 25, 232

Durbin, Dick 129–30

E

Edwards, John 89

Eli Lilly 10

Emord, Jonathan 122–23, 257

energy healing 187-93, 269

energy psychology techniques 80, 248

emotions 62, 63-4, 74, 76, 82-3, 106, 242, 246

epidemics 166, 172, 221–22

epilepsy 40

European Union's Food Supplements Directive (FSD) 132–36,

138, 258
Every-Palmer, Susanna 8–9, 228, 230
evidence-based medicine (EBM) 7–8
exercise 2, 10, 32, 45, 63, 65, 69, 96–7, 104, 106, 109, 161–69, 184–
    85, 207, 217, 223, 243–44, 263–65, 275
  exercise program 45, 97, 165, 167–68
  exercise therapy 164, 264
eye movement desensitization and reprocessing (EMDR) 77–80,
    246–48

F

failed back surgery syndrome (FBSS) 51–2
FDA 25, 123, 129, 196, 216, 257
fertility 146, 200
feverfew 154, 261
fibromyalgia 41, 47, 67, 72, 75, 80, 81, 82, 84, 98, 104–05, 115,
    118–19, 162, 164–67, 178–79, 184–85, 199, 237–38, 245, 247–
    48, 253, 257, 264–65, 268, 269
  fibromyalgia patients 75, 105, 119, 167, 245, 268
  fibromyalgia sufferers 72, 184
  fibromyalgia symptoms 185
flavonoids 112
flaxseed 121
food 2, 10, 63, 112, 114, 122, 127–28, 132–42, 174, 229
  dairy 120
  food containing gluten 142
  food safety 137, 139, 141
  food sensitivities 2, 142
  food supplements 132, 133, 135, 138, 140
frankincense 151, 259
Roosevelt, Franklin, D. 167, 265

G

gastrointestinal 34, 35, 38, 142, 155–56, 158, 206, 235
  gastritis 35
  gastroenterological 245
  gastrointestinal complications 34, 235
  gastrointestinal symptoms 142
Gause, Valerie 215
ginger 154, 155, 261
Glaxosmithkline 10, 229
glucosamine and chondroitin 156–59, 262, 263
gluten 142–45
  gluten-free 144
government 11, 12, 14, 20, 29, 38, 85, 90, 122, 129, 130, 134, 196,
  203, 250
grapefruit 112
grapeseed 113
Graves, James 28–9
Grazione, John 100–01, 279
green tea 155
Gronowicz, Gloria 188–91
Gussenhoven, Rob 30
gynecological 154

H

hallucinations 197
harm 11, 12, 42, 84, 130, 189, 221, 273–74
  harm reduction 273–74
headaches 10, 41, 62, 67–8, 71, 72, 73, 80, 81, 87, 88, 115, 154,
  178, 184, 195, 245, 246, 247, 255
health claims 122, 123, 127, 131, 139, 140
health coach 121
health food 141, 174
health insurance 2, 86, 105, 213, 222
health organization 88, 112, 140, 149, 185, 269

heartburn 21
hematology 27
hemorrhage 34
hepatotoxicity 37, 236
herbs 2, 8, 12, 36, 127, 132, 149–51, 155, 260
   herbal medicines 150, 259
   herbal remedies 150, 259, 261
   herbal treatments 149, 151, 153, 155, 157, 159, 259
herniated disc 55–7
Hoffman, Philip Seymour 22, 285
holistic 36, 118, 279
   holistic physician 118, 279
homeopathy 11, 171–79, 187, 223, 266–68
   homeopathic hospitals 175
   homeopathic physician 174
   homeopathic remedies 171, 173–74
   homeopathic treatment 178, 179
hospital 43, 89–90, 99, 100, 162, 173, 176–77, 185, 193, 213, 267, 270, 278
Howick, Jeremy 8, 9, 228, 230
hydrochloride 157, 233
hydrocodone 17, 22, 26, 31, 234
hyperalgesia 30, 234
hypnosis 61, 82–4, 249
hypoglycemia 34
Hysingla ER 26

I

ibuprofen 17, 31, 33–6, 38–9, 58, 156, 206, 235, 262
immune 30, 37, 63, 115, 121, 142–43, 198, 210, 234
   immune disorders 115
   immune response 63
   immune suppression 234

immune system 30, 37, 121, 142–43
immunosuppression 201, 234
industry 89, 125, 127, 130, 136, 227, 252
inflammation 2, 33, 38, 40, 42, 69, 111–13, 116, 151, 155, 199,
   201, 209, 214, 261, 275
   inflammation research 261
   inflammatory 113, 151, 174, 255
ingredients 111, 127–29, 131, 133–34, 140, 149
integrative medicine 230, 248–49, 253, 269
integrative pain 252, 254, 259, 265, 268
interdisciplinary 45, 46, 93, 108, 217–18, 278
intervention 8, 11–12, 51, 58, 74, 81, 85, 103, 157, 186, 239, 243–
   45, 276
ischemia 108

J

Jackson, Michael 21, 232, 285
Johns Hopkins 20, 46, 227
Johnson & Johnson 10, 229–30, 276
joint pain 41, 58, 113, 115, 142–44, 146
juicing 36, 121

K

Kelleher, Michelle 100, 279
Kennedy, John F. 163, 264
kidney 34, 38
   kidney failure 34
   kidney insufficiency 34
kinesiophobia 162, 263
knee 21, 40, 51, 58–9, 98, 117, 151, 153, 156–57, 165, 184, 205,
   241–42, 253, 256, 260–63, 265
   knee osteoarthritis 156–57, 184, 262–63, 265

knee pain 51, 58, 98, 117, 153, 205, 263
knee surgery 58
Kolodny, Andrew 23, 232
Kong, Philomena 185–86, 279
Kraus-Weber 45, 162–64

L

laboratory 128, 188, 189, 211
LaGuardia Report 195–96
laser therapy 50, 178, 209-16, 275-77
laughter 61, 243
laws 25, 28, 131, 135, 202, 203, 204, 274
legalize 182, 196
  legalize acupuncture 182
  legalize medical marijuana 196
legislation 132, 133, 139, 141, 196, 221-25
leukemia 69, 201
Levine, Peter 62, 76
Leyden, Martin 70, 279
lidocaine 43, 45
Lizzi, Frank 27–8
low-back pain 18, 25–6, 51, 52, 55–6, 62, 64, 67, 88, 98, 103–04, 118, 147, 158, 162, 164, 166–69, 179, 184, 186, 231, 239, 240–44, 251, 252, 253, 256, 263–64, 265–66, 268–69, 277–78

M

magnesium 111, 118–19, 133, 256–57
magnetic resonance imaging (MRI) 2, 55–6, 94–5, 119–20, 239
mainstream medical 14, 188
malnourished 37
  malnutrition 142
manipulative and body-based practices 89, 91, 93, 95, 97, 99, 101,

103, 105, 107, 109, 249
manslaughter 21, 28
manual therapy 96, 252-53
Marcus, Norman 44–50, 238, 241–42, 247, 259, 263–64, 279
Maroon, Joseph 113, 254
Marrone, Dick 99, 279
Mayo Clinic 13, 255
marijuana 150, 195–207, 270, 271–73, 274–75
  marijuana dispensaries 204, 275
  marijuana seized 200, 272
  marijuana, gateway 202, 273
Maryland 46, 249
Massachusetts 13, 24
massage 12, 36, 46, 49, 96-8, 101-07, 186, 216, 223-24, 252-53, 269
Masterson, Lee 92–3, 250, 279
medication 10, 22, 26–7, 31, 35–6, 56, 71, 72, 94, 103, 114, 146, 168, 185, 195, 204, 214, 217
Medtronics 54
menstrual 195
mental health 32, 33, 71, 81, 85–6, 108, 202, 222, 224, 249
  mental disorders 14
  mental illness 85, 201
Mercola, Joseph 118, 254–56, 279
Mesmer, Anton 84
migraine 41, 67, 68, 71, 73, 80, 84, 152–54, 178–79, 195, 245–47, 260–61, 267
miscarriage 154
Moertel, Charles 13
Mount Sinai Medical School 84
morphine 17, 30, 185, 202, 239, 274
Murray, Conrad 21

N

naloxone 25, 233

naproxen 17, 36
narcotics 17, 24, 29, 56, 59, 116, 195, 217, 233
  narcotics manufacturers 24
  narcotics makers 233
National Academy of Sciences 1
neck pain 1, 59, 62, 67, 87–8, 103, 107, 164, 184, 210, 211, 216, 264, 276
neuralgia 41, 210, 275
neurofeedback 14–15, 67, 72–3, 108, 245–46
Neurontin 17, 40–2
neuropathic 80, 117–18, 197, 199, 212, 237, 256, 262, 272
neuroscience 243, 245–46
Nexium 35
NSAIDs 17, 18, 33–6, 38–9, 88, 104, 113, 152, 155–56, 174, 211, 255, 260
numbness 43, 57, 117, 142
Nutrasweet 142, 145

O

ointment 174, 266
Oklahoma 182
omega-3 fatty acids 111, 112–13, 254
opioids 17, 18–20, 23–6, 28, 30–3, 111, 202, 214, 221, 231–35, 254, 274
  opioid addiction 18, 23, 33
  opioid agonist 25
  opioid overdose 19, 202, 214
  opioid prescribing 23, 32, 231, 235
  opioid therapy 30, 32, 111, 234, 254
osteoarthritis 35, 51, 58, 84, 103, 115, 151, 153–58, 163, 165, 174, 178–79, 184, 210, 241, 242, 253, 256, 260–65, 268
oxycodone 11, 17, 22, 25, 233
oxycontin 11, 20, 25, 218, 232

P

pain conditions 1, 41, 47, 67, 162, 211
pain education 3, 68, 227
pain management 3, 5, 18, 22, 28, 46, 61, 79, 84, 100, 102, 120, 150, 217, 219, 224, 227–28, 232, 247, 249, 252, 254, 259, 265, 266, 268, 269, 275, 278
pain medicine 11, 31, 228, 232 –39, 245, 247–48, 251–52, 254, 259, 268, 278
Pain Treatment Parity Act 221-25
painkillers 19, 21–4, 28, 30, 37, 58, 63, 210, 221, 233, 235
pancreatitis 34
paralysis 44, 49, 95, 167
Paxil 9, 21
Pauling, Linus 13, 15
Pennebaker, James 75–6, 246
Pershing, Steven 214–15
pharmaceuticals 2, 10, 11, 14, 16–17, 20, 122, 127, 132, 149, 187, 236
Phillips, Maggie 62
physical therapy 27, 32, 36, 45, 50, 57-8, 84, 96-101, 104, 119-20, 158, 164, 184, 186, 211, 217, 251-53, 264
Pittsburgh 113
placebo 8–9, 39, 41, 44, 58, 117, 153–54, 157, 158, 175, 178–79, 184, 211–12, 242, 260, 267–69
plasma 44, 207, 243
policy 25, 29, 88, 195, 228, 249, 250, 251
post-traumatic stress disorder (PTSD) 13–14, 22, 77–8, 80–1, 246.
prediabetic 120–21
Primary Care Trusts 175
Prozac 9, 14
psychological factors 52, 53–4
psychosis 200, 273
Purdue Pharmaceuticals 11, 20, 26, 232

Q

quantitative EEG (QEEG) 73

R

Rackauckas, Tony 25
RAND Corporation 87
randomized controlled trials 43, 154, 156
randomized placebo-controlled trials 261
randomized clinical trials 7, 168, 211, 266
randomized controlled study 72, 81, 103, 104, 113, 117–18, 149, 156, 174, 244
Rappaport, Rob 25
regulations 127, 128, 139, 258, 259
rehabilitation 3, 31, 93, 97, 102, 166, 185, 217, 241, 244, 264–66, 277
Reiki 187, 192-93
Reston, James 182, 268
Reuben, Scott 11
rheumatism 151, 195
rheumatoid arthritis 113, 145, 153, 156, 163, 165, 178, 199, 237, 255, 267
Rolf, Ida 105
rolfing 102, 105–07, 253–54
Rosa, Emily 191–92

S

Sarno, John 74–5, 246
Saul, Andrew 14–15, 230, 279
sciatica 88, 169, 239, 266

sedative 21, 150
seizures 34, 40, 132
Shapiro, Francine 77–78, 246–47
specialists 23, 24, 27, 33, 56
SSRIs 9, 17, 228
steroids 17, 33, 40, 43, 114, 211
stillbirths 34
Structural Integration 102, 105, 107, 253-54
sugar 8, 112, 146, 156, 259
surgery 2, 18, 21, 43, 46, 48–9 , 51–9, 65, 92, 95–6, 105, 120, 121, 155, 164, 182, 186–88, 214, 216, 218, 231, 238–42, 244, 262, 275, 278

T

Taarborrelli, Randy 21
Targaniq ER 25
Taskin, Donald 201
Taylor, Doyle 89
technology 20, 24, 52, 66, 89, 213, 244, 250
tendonitis 210
Tennessee 214
tension 2, 45, 61, 62, 66–8, 70, 71, 74, 161, 245
Therapeutic Touch 187, 189, 191-93, 269-70
therapists 96–7, 99, 100–102, 104, 186, 222, 224, 252, 269
tobacco 147
trauma 2, 13, 14, 22, 53, 61–3, 74, 76–8, 107, 240
tricyclics 17
turmeric 155, 262
Tylenol 33, 37, 48, 206

U

ulcers 35, 214
ultrasound 96, 97, 119

UN Global Impact Fund 213
United States Pharmacopeia 195
US Bureau of Labor Statistics 99, 250, 252

V

vaccinations 38, 131, 236
valium 22
Van der Kolk, Bessel 13–14, 230
Verkerk, Robert 124–26, 133–34, 137–39, 279
Vermont 24, 100
vertebrae 42, 57, 95
Vicodin 21, 31, 47
Vioxx 38, 39, 236
vitamins 13, 47, 109, 111, 112–18, 124–27, 134, 136–38, 141, 255–
56, 260

W

warnings 26, 35, 36, 44, 54, 75, 129, 154
Wellstone, Paul 222
West Virginia 19
World Federation of Chiropractic 88
World Health Organization (WHO) 88, 140, 149, 185, 269
Wyoming 182

X

x-rays 95, 119, 163
Xanax 21, 22

Y

YMCA 163, 164, 168
yoga 168–69, 265, 266

Z

Zoloft 21
Zohydro 24, 25, 122, 233–34